ANIMAL PAIN

A PRACTICE-ORIENTED APPROACH
TO AN EFFECTIVE PAIN CONTROL
IN ANIMALS

Edited by

Ludo J. Hellebrekers
Faculty of Veterinary Medicine,
University of Utrecht, The Netherlands

cw · VAN DER WEES · uitgeverij
Utrecht, The Netherlands, 2000

ISBN 90 5805 030 0
NUGI 749

Design by Roel Venderbosch, Wychen
Typeset by Alces alces, Utrecht
Printed by Hentenaar boek, Nieuwegein

Publisher:
cv · **VAN DER WEES** · *uitgeverij*
Janskerkhof 26
3512 BN Utrecht
The Netherlands
t (+) 31 (0) 30 231 43 21
f (+) 31 (0) 30 231 08 60
e vdwees@xs4all.nl

TABLE OF CONTENTS

CONTRIBUTORS

Nienke Endenburg, PhD
Faculty of Veterinary Medicine, Utrecht University,
Utrecht, The Netherlands

Elizabeth M. Hardie, DVM, PhD, DipACVS
College of Veterinary Medicine, North Carolina State University,
Raleigh, NC, USA

Ludo J. Hellebrekers, DVM, PhD, DipECVA
Faculty of Veterinary Medicine, Utrecht University,
Utrecht, The Netherlands

B Duncan X Lascelles, BSc BVSc PhD MRCVS CertVA DSAS(Soft Tissue)
DipECVS
Department of Clinical Veterinary Science, University of Bristol,
Langford House, Langford, UK

Karol A. Mathews
Ontario Veterinary College, University of Guelph, Guelph,
Canada

Sharon Redrobe BSc(Hons) BVetMed CertLAS MRCVS
Bristol Zoo Gardens, Clifton, Bristol, UK

Bernard E. Rollin, PhD
Director of Bioethical Planning, Colorado State University,
Fort Collins, CO, USA

Urs Schatzmann, DVM, PhD, DipECVA
Klinik für Nutztiere und Pferde der Universität Bern, Bern,
Switzerland

PREFACE

"Pain is an emotion that dwells in the brain"
(Plato, ca. 375 BC)

The International Association for the Study of Pain (IASP) has defined pain as "the unpleasant sensory and/or emotional experience associated with actual or potential tissue damage". This definition, although set forth for the human patient, is now uniformly applied to animals subjected to a nociceptive, or painful, stimulation as well. It is only in the latter decades of the last century that mankind has come to recognise that animals can be subject to painful experiences, where in former times the violent struggle and vocalisation seen during or after surgical intervention were interpreted as being autonomic nervous system responses or uncontrolled muscular reflexes.

At the beginning of the 21st century, there is a large body of basic knowledge of, and insight into, neuroanatomical and neuro-physiological characteristics in man and animal alike, as well as a rapidly enlarging understanding of pain physiology. Together, this has come to support the view that animals record, transport, process and modulate nociceptive signals in a fashion similar to man. It has now become generally accepted that, despite the lack of possibility for verbal communication concerning this painful stimulation, animals undergo an 'unpleasant experience' in circumstances similar to those in humans, in this regard.

Research in laboratory animals as well as experience in human neonates has unequivocally shown that the young individual's pain perception is stronger rather than less than that in adults, and that a short-duration procedure with a high pain intensity will result in an 'unpleasant experience' that long outlasts the initial period of stimulation.

Taking into account all the above, pain control in animals remains a matter of great concern, especially considering the fact that less then half of the canine patients are routinely treated with analgesic medication, post-surgically.

Looking at other species following surgery, the percentage of animals that go untreated rises rapidly when we look at cats, horses, or other species.

It can be stated that, in general, the veterinarian's knowledge regarding background pathophysiology, options for analgesic therapy and limitations due to negative side effects, might indeed be limited. This is especially true with regard to the less common animal species.

Presently there is an obvious awareness of the (potential) presence of pain and its negative consequence for the animal's well being and overall health status. This puts a clear responsibility on veterinarians to try to achieve adequate pain relief in the animals entrusted to their care.

Nowadays, veterinarians also need to get actively involved in the discussion about so called 'minor' surgical procedures that, up to the present day, are still performed without any analgesic support whatsoever, based on an argument of business economics, relatively short duration of the procedure or (under)developmental state of the neurological system.

The authors expect this book to provide the reader with the tools to more effectively achieve adequate pain relief in animals, and feel that it will also supply relevant arguments in support of the 'added value' of adequate pain relief both for the animal and for the animal's owner.

Ludo J. Hellebrekers, editor
Utrecht, The Netherlands
Spring 2000

1

PAIN IN ANIMALS

Ludo J. Hellebrekers, DVM, PhD, DipECVA,
Faculty of Veterinary Medicine, Utrecht University, Utrecht,
The Netherlands

In recent years, both within the veterinary profession as well as in society as a whole, increasing attention has been focussed on the problems of pain in animals — its recognition, alleviation and subsequent prevention.

When we consider the phenomenon of 'pain in animals' a number of questions arise:
- *does pain actually occur in animals?*
- *to what extent is the presence of pain detrimental to the health and/or well-being of the animal?*
- *how can pain in animals be recognised and subsequently quantified?*
- *what options do we have available to effectively alleviate pain in animals?*

Does pain actually occur in animals?

In the past, animals were generally considered to be of a lower developmental or evolutionary level than man, and as a consequence were thought not to possess any sensation of pain, as mankind knew it. This view in itself did not preclude the observation that, when an animal was wounded, it would respond with violent movements, loud vocalisation and aversive behaviour. However, these observations were at that time 'determined' to be autonomous nervous system phenomena rather than a conscious response to an 'unpleasant sensory sensation'.

Although some may find these observations hard to accept, it has to be realised that although we now have the knowledge that allows us to better understand pain physiology in animals and man, and allows us to accept the fact that animals can indeed experience pain, we do not always apply this knowledge in a consistent fashion. Examples of this are abundantly present all around us and include surgical interventions in commercially kept animals, such as beak trimming in baby chicks and the docking and castration of piglets, all done without any form of anaesthesia or pain control. Similarly, in the companion animal sector, the same animals that are kept and cared for as 'family members' are being surgically treated by the removal of dew claws, tail docking or ear cropping (although some of these procedures are now forbidden by law in some countries) without any form of anaesthesia or analgesia applied.

The argument used to justify these procedures centres on the aspect that these interventions usually take place in the period shortly (< 3 weeks) after birth and/or that the duration of the intervention is very short. The argument in support of these interventions being executed at a very young age is based upon the belief that at that stage in life the nervous system, ultimately responsible for the recognition and processing of the pain stimuli, is still not fully developed. This would prevent (conscious) sensation of stimuli determined to be painful in later life.

It is exactly this view regarding the functioning of the nervous system in neonates that was upheld in human anaesthesiology for a long time. This resulted in a situation whereby human neonates, all through the 1970s and early 1980s, underwent minor surgical procedures without any form of pain relief. Research performed since then has unequivocally proven that even very young babies can also experience pain [1] and that, for instance, the vocalisation during the intervention in unanaesthetised babies can be clearly differentiated from other forms of (non pain-related) crying.

Considering the above, it remains surprising that most people still consider the vocalisation of puppies during tail docking or the (vocal) response of piglets during castration to be primarily related to the (temporary) separation from the mother, rather then to ascribe this response to the intense injury- or surgery-induced pain.

Both the behavioural response patterns as well as numerous other changes (physiological, biochemical) support the view that even at a very young age, animals just like humans can experience pain as an 'unpleasant sensation'.

The question remains: What evidence do we have for the statement that animals undergo pain as an 'unpleasant sensory or emotional experience'? When we consider the anatomy of the central nervous system, with the organisation of the brain, the spinal cord and the peripheral nervous system network, together with its neuro-physiological characteristics, there are great similarities between man and animals. The major difference lies in the fact that humans, contrary to animals, can relate their pain experience verbally. Despite the fact that animals cannot verbally relate their painful experience, it is now generally accepted that animals do in fact experience pain. Research has shown that many of the (quantifiable) response patterns of animals to pain stimuli are similar to those occurring in humans experiencing painful situations. In both man and animals, the heart rate increases, a (temporary) hypertension occurs and the changes in plasma levels of the different stress hormones demonstrate similar patterns.

Based upon the above, it can no longer be considered acceptable that bodily harm is intentionally inflicted onto animals without anaesthesia or (pre-, per- or post-operative) analgesia. In this respect any form of surgical intervention can be seen as 'purposeful bodily harm' with a certain amount of pain, the extent of which depends on the type and severity of the intervention.

A major problem remains in the recognition and subsequent quantification of pain behaviour in animals. This problem is for a substantial part due to the fact that the different animal species exhibit their behavioural patterns, and specifically those related to or induced by pain, in distinctly different ways. Just consider the difference between species such as dogs and cats in the way they respond to painful stimuli in their respective ways. In general, dogs will respond favourably to extra attention from humans in their environment while most cats will turn away from humans, to be left to their own resources. Interpretation becomes even more troublesome when we are working with animal species of which the normal behavioural patterns are even less familiar to us (such as rabbits or rodents) or when the situation involves animal species that are primarily kept commercially within the agricultural sector, such as cattle or swine.

In order to prevent animal suffering from going unrecognised, and consequently untreated, it has been long-term practice in the animal research world to apply the *Principle of Analogy*. The basis of this principle lies in the assumption that those (surgical) interventions that are known to be painful in humans are considered to be painful in animals as well. When this principle is applied in the decision making regarding the development of an anaesthetic or analgesic protocol, it is the animal that gets 'the benefit of the doubt' and as a consequence, upon recognition of the presence of pain, the realisation of adequate pain relief is mandatory.

What are the negative aspects of pain in animals?

Next to the fact that, similar to the situation in humans, overall welfare is impaired when animals are experiencing (post-operative) pain, a number of specific negative aspects can be recognised:

- *through activation of the stress response wound healing will be impaired*
- *on account of the increased energy consumption and decreased food (energy) intake the animals are more easily prone to a negative energy-balance*
- *there is increased incidence of delayed recovery post-anaesthesia and a greater risk of post-operative complications*
- *respiration will become less efficient*
- *the risk for auto-mutilation and biting on wounds increases*
- *with a prolonged period of pain, the pain may become chronic in character and thereby more difficult to treat*
- *on account of the prolonged stress, the body's overall resistance to infections diminishes, increasing the incidence of complications.*

An argument often used against the application of pain treatment is that, for instance, under circumstances of an injured leg, it is the pain that prevents the animal from putting weight on the leg thereby preventing further damage. There is no doubt that by showing signs of pain (i.e. limping due to an injured leg) the attention of the owner or caretaker of the animal is drawn to the problem, while at the same time the absence of weight bearing promotes the early stages of the healing process. Despite this, adequate pain control following a properly conducted surgical intervention can only support a fast and uncomplicated recovery. Research has shown that a proper post-operative pain protocol promotes the quality of the recovery and is beneficial for the wound healing. The animal will resume a normal eating pattern and loose less weight than those without adequate pain control.

How to recognise pain in animals?

As stated before, the recognition and quantification of pain in animals remains a difficult and sometimes hazardous task under the best of circumstances. However, based upon the *Principle of Analogy*, it should prove possible to make an estimation of the level of pain and discomfort under specific circumstances. Most animal owners, especially those of animals such as dogs, cats and horses, are more than able to detect behavioural changes in their animals and thus provide an indication for the presence of pain or discomfort. The practising veterinarian is in a much more difficult situation. Not only is he or she, when compared to the owner, much less acquainted with the individual animal in question, but also the animal's behaviour will usually also be strongly influenced by the 'strange' and potentially threatening surroundings of the veterinary practice.

As a result of these factors, the animal will demonstrate signs of pain less clearly, and a detailed description of the behavioural changes observed by the owner can be very helpful in establishing the diagnosis of pain.

How can pain in animals be effectively alleviated?

In order to effectively alleviate pain in animals a detailed knowledge of pain physiology, including the different pain pathways, the (chemical) mediators and receptor types involved, is needed. Only then can the different types of pain treatment protocols be optimally employed to obtain a maximal pain relief.

It is these and other topics that will discussed throughout this book. It will provide a comprehensive overview of not only the practical aspects of pain relief in different categories of animal species, but also supply relevant information on the ethical, physiological and pharmacological background that provide the basis for such therapy.

Selected bibliography

1 Fitzgerald M. Pain and analgesia in neonates. Trends in Neuroscience 1987;10:344.
2 Fitzgerald M. Neurobiology of foetal and neonatal pain. In: Textbook of Pain, (3rd edn), Wall P, Melzack R (Eds), Churchill Livingstone, London 1994:153-63.
3 Lascelles BDX. Advances in the control of pain in animals. Veterinary Annual 1996:1-15.
4 Wall PD. Defining pain in animals. In: Short CE, Van Poznak A (Eds), Animal Pain, Churchill Livingstone, Edinburgh 1992:62.

2

THE ETHICS OF PAIN CONTROL IN COMPANION ANIMALS

Bernard E. Rollin, *PhD*, *Professor of Philosophy*,
Professor of Physiology, *Director of Bioethical Planning*,
Colorado State University, Fort Collins, CO, USA

The rise of new social ethics for animals

No one at all attentive to social change can doubt that western societies in Europe, North America, Australia, and New Zealand have been developing significant ethical concern for animal treatment in the course of the last three decades. Most evident, perhaps, are the laws and policies that have been adopted protecting the interests of research animals in such countries as Great Britain, the US, the Netherlands, Sweden, Australia, New Zealand, Switzerland, and Germany, all aimed at minimising animal pain and suffering. Indeed, in the US in 1985, two sets of laws serving this end were adopted, despite explicit and widely publicised threats from the medical research community that any constraints on animal use would endanger human health. Whereas in the US 20 years ago one would have found virtually no legislation pending related to animal protection in federal, state or local legislatures, such bills have now proliferated, ranging in scope from laws abolishing rodeos, to referendums abolishing the steel-jawed trap and spring bear hunts, to laws making the slaughter of horses for food a felony. According to the executive director of the largest equine organisation in the United States, the bills pertaining to horse welfare alone proposed in the US in 1998 comprised a volume as thick as a large city telephone book (personal communication).

Indeed, according to both the National Institutes of Health and National Cattlemen's Association, neither of whom have a vested interest in over-inflating the influence of social concerns for animals, the US Congress has received more letters, faxes, phone calls and personal contacts regarding animal issues than on any other matters.

The treatment of agricultural animals in industrialised agriculture has become a major priority in Europe, with Sweden passing legislation in 1988 abolishing confinement agriculture and creating what the New York Times called 'a bill of rights for farm animals'. Similar rules have been promulgated in Britain, and farm animal welfare is a major priority for the EC. Furthermore, according to a very plausible interpretation of results obtained by George Gaskell and his associates, moral concern for animals probably weighs very heavily, and possibly more heavily than fear of risk, in European rejection of biotechnology [1].

Such dramatic changes in social ethics require explanation, in virtue of the fact that moral theory and practice pertaining to animals was virtually non-existent throughout most of human history. The one exception was the prohibition of deliberate cruelty to animals, that is, deliberate, purposeless, willful, deviant, sadistic, or intentional infliction of pain and suffering or egregious neglect upon animals. While legal expression of this prohibition may be found even in the Bible and in virtually all civilised societies, it affords only minimal protection for animals. For one thing, as legal theory and practice attest, the anti-cruelty laws spring in part from anthropocentric considerations, that is, the realization that those who commit such acts on animals will inexorably move to similar behaviour towards people — an ancient insight borne out by modern research. Second, these laws do not apply to standard animal uses. Thus, no scientific research performed in a university can ever be actionable under the cruelty laws, no matter how much pain or suffering it produces. This is equally true of agricultural practices, rodeo, hunting, trapping or any other non-deviant animal use. Third, given over-crowded courts and jails, these laws are rarely enforced.

The minimalistic nature of the anti-cruelty ethic may be made manifest by the following thought experiment. Consider a pie chart representing all of the suffering that animals experience at human hands, and ask yourself what percentage of that suffering results from deliberate cruelty. Every audience I have ever addressed on this subject says the same things: 'A tiny slice', 'only 1%'. When we realise that the US alone produces 8 billion broiler chickens per year in confinement, and 80% of these animals go to market with fractures or deep bone bruises, we realise the wisdom of the audience response. So we can now characterise the nature of the socio-ethical revolution regarding animal treatment that we have been discussing: in essence, society has started to worry about the 99+% of animal suffering that is *not* the result of deliberate cruelty.

Why has this new concern arisen during the last three decades? Firstly, because of changes in social demography. Western societies have become increasingly urban and suburban. In the US, only 1.5% of the population is engaged in production agriculture, with probably a third of that small percentage in animal agriculture. This in turn means that the paradigm for an animal in the social mind has changed from the cow or horse of a hundred years ago — food animal or beast of burden — to the companion animal or pet, the dog or cat most of society professes to see as 'a member of the family'. Second, the mass media have discovered that 'animal concerns sell papers' and that the public never tires of animal stories. Thus, animal abuse and suffering is ubiquitously publicised.

Third, the public has gradually become aware that the nature of animal use has changed precipitously and dramatically since World War II. Although both historically and today animal agriculture — the use of animals for food, fibre, locomotion and power — has been the predominant use of animals in society, the nature of animal agriculture has undergone a major metamorphosis. Before 1950, the key to successful animal agriculture was husbandry, a term derived from the old Norse word for 'bonded to the household'. This meant placing the animals into the optimal environment for which they were suited biologically and then augmenting their natural ability to survive by human provision of protection from predators, medical attention, food and water during famine and drought respectively, and so on. This has been called the ancient and fair contract between humans and animals, with both parties better off in virtue of the relationship. So powerful is this metaphor in the human psyche, in fact, that when the Psalmist wishes to provide a metaphor for God's ideal relationship to humans, he chooses the shepherd: 'The Lord is my shepherd, I shall not want'. Husbandry agriculture, then, was about putting square pegs into square holes, round pegs in round holes, and creating as little friction as possible in doing so.

All of this changed in the mid-twentieth century with industrialised agriculture. Industry replaced husbandry, efficiency and productivity eclipsed care. With the advent of 'technological sanders', such as antibiotics and vaccines, we could force square pegs into round holes and keep animals in environments where they suffered, yet continued to be productive. Similarly, the post-World War II rise of large amounts of animal research and testing also did not qualify as a fair contract comparable to husbandry: we hurt animals, inflicted upon them disease, fear, stress, etc. in ways that benefitted us, but which provided no compensatory benefit to the animal subjects. As society has become aware of these new, unfair uses of animals, it has groped for language to express its moral concern that, if we use animals, we treat them fairly as we did in traditional husbandry.

Fourth, a significant number of scientists and philosophers have helped society articulate a new ethic for animals — Peter Singer, Tom Regan, Bernard Rollin, Steve Sapontzis, Jane Goodall. Though there are marked differences among all of these philosophical approaches, there is a strong common central core. Most important, all agree that an ethic of anticruelty, and laws reflecting that ethic, do not morally suffice. Society must address and eliminate as much as possible animal pain and suffering in its animal use and must elevate the moral and legal status of animals.

Fifth, society was ready to think ethically about animals, having spent decades shining an ethical searchlight on the treatment of traditionally disenfranchised humans — women, blacks and other minorities, the disabled, third world residents and even the environment. Further, many of the people advocating higher moral status for animals were veterans of other moral crusades, such as civil rights, the labour movement, the women's movement, and so on.

Deriving a new ethic for animals

The core of philosophical arguments aimed at raising the moral status of animals is not difficult to articulate. When it became manifest that the traditional ethic for animals, the prohibition against cruelty, was conceptually incapable of capturing most animal uses and the attendant suffering they occasioned, it was clear that an augmented set of ethical concepts was required. But, as Plato pointed out long ago, one does not create ethical concepts *ex nihilo*. Whether one is dealing with other individuals or with society in general, in an attempt to change their ethical thinking, one cannot simply force new ethical ideas on others. In Plato's judicious locution, when one is attempting to persuade adults of the necessity of changing their ethical positions, one cannot *teach*, one must instead *remind*. Whereas in the case of factual information, such as the capital cities of foreign countries or the parasites that infect dogs, one can certainly teach from personal expertise in the empirically based area, no one enjoys unique expertise in matters of right and wrong in the same way, since ethical judgments are not validated by empirical methods. If I wish to convince you of an ethical position, the most sensible strategy is to show you that the position I am defending is *already implicit in what you believe*, but you have not gone through the requisite reasoning to become aware of it. By leading you to that reasoning I prompt you to 'recollect' what you have failed to notice.

An excellent example of such a move may be found in the US in Lyndon Johnson's approach to the ethical principles underlying civil rights legislation. As he was a Southerner himself, Johnson realised that most Southerners would acquiesce to the following two assumptions:
- *all humans should be treated equally and*
- *blacks are humans.*

The problem was that they had never been 'reminded' to draw the conclusion entailed by those assumptions, namely:

Blacks should be treated equally.

Johnson saw that embodying these ideas in law would make people 'recollect', and he was right.

In my own metaphor, paralleling Plato's, those who would change the ethics of another must use judo (a person's own force against them), not sumo (your force against theirs). The above mentioned civil rights example does precisely this, a point especially manifest when one compares it with an example of sumo, or teaching rather than reminding, in twentieth century American history. I am referring to Prohibition, wherein a small group of individuals, and certainly a minority, attempted to force the majority to stop drinking. Not only did the law not work, people actually drank *more*. If President Johnson had been wrong about being able to remind or use 'judo' to get people to see that equal rights followed from their own beliefs, the Civil Rights legislation would have been as socially meaningless and stillborn as Prohibition.

Thus if people are seeking to supplant the traditional, limited anti-cruelty ethic for animals with a more substantive set of moral principles, they must heed Plato's principle, and this is indeed what has occurred. People have looked to our social consensus ethic for *humans* as articulated in Western democratic societies and attempted to apply it, *mutatis mutandis* (i.e., appropriately modified), to animal treatment, even as that same ethic has been gradually expanded to include women, children, minorities, the handicapped, etc.

Philosophically, the key to expanding the application of that ethic to animals or to disenfranchised humans is demonstrating that there are most of all no *morally relevant differences* between those to whom the ethical machinery is being fully applied and those who have been excluded from its purview. This task has been successfully prosecuted by a number of philosophers during the past three decades [2-5]. Though their arguments differ in details, all of these philosophers have shown that there are no morally relevant reasons for excluding animals from the application of our ethical machinery to an assessment of their treatment. For example, some have argued that we can do whatever we wish to animals because we are more powerful than they are. It is easy to see that such reasoning, if accepted, would serve to justify the actions of murderers, rapists, muggers, and tyrants, and would vitiate morality altogether, for it entails an acceptance of 'might makes right'.

All other attempts to exclude animals from the moral arena on the basis of alleged morally relevant differences between them and us can be shown to be equally unworkable [3]. Such moves include claiming that humans have souls and animals do not, that humans are evolutionarily superior, that humans are rational and animals are not, that animals are not conscious or capable of experiencing morally relevant mental states, that morality arises out of contract among rational human beings, and so on. All of the above can be easily countered, at least to the satisfaction of society in general.

It does not, of course, suffice to show that there are no morally relevant reasons for excluding animals from consideration by our full moral machinery. One must also show that there are positive, morally relevant similarities for including them. Fortunately, this too is manifest to common sense. In democratic societies we strike a balance between the good of human individuals and the good of society or the group by building protective fences around fundamental aspects of human nature to protect those basic interests *even* from the general welfare. Freedom of speech, freedom of belief, protection from torture, holding on to one's property are all encoded as *moral/legal rights* designed to protect what is essential to human nature from encroachment for the sake of general benefit. It has become clear that animals too have natures, what Aristotle called *telos*, the 'cowness' of the cow, the 'pigness' of the pig. Indeed, traditional animal use in agriculture could not succeed without respecting those natures; in fact, meeting the needs that flowed from those natures was the essence of *animal husbandry*-based agriculture, with failure to respect those natures harming the farmer as much as the animal through diminished productivity. Unfortunately, modern industrialised intensive agriculture allows us to ignore the animals' natures or *teloi* and force square pegs into round holes by use of technological sanders such as antibiotics and vaccines. Animal research, too, is a relatively new animal use that often involves violating animal natures, if only in how the animals are kept.

The concept of guaranteed legal protection for basic animal needs and natures is surely one of the fundamental moral insights underlying the revolutionary changes we discussed earlier in this paper. It is of course most obviously instantiated in the aforementioned Swedish law abolishing confinement agriculture failing to respect the animals' *telos*, but it conceptually undergirds virtually all of the many pieces of legislation being proposed and passed on national and local levels to protect animals.

Barriers to actualizing the New Ethic

However well-intentioned society may be regarding the moral status of animals, there is manifestly a fundamental conceptual barrier to achieving full moral recognition for them and their interests. This barrier stems, of course, from the fact that society seems to be unwilling to abandon the benefits that emerge from major areas of animal use, though it does seem to be moving towards eliminating areas of animal use perceived as frivolous or outrageous. Examples falling under these latter categories include testing cosmetics on animals, some forms of hunting and trapping, some forms of animal shows, perhaps some military uses, and certain forms of agricultural production systems. But on the other hand, society seems to fully accept in principle the use of animals for food and fibre, and for advancing medical knowledge and treatment modalities.

This mind-set naturally puts a limit on the extension of our ethic for humans to animals. Most obviously, the killing of animals for food is largely unquestioned, except insofar as slaughter generates pain, fear, and suffering. Similarly, not only is the painless killing of animals for biomedical research accepted, so too is some element of pain and suffering if the nature of the research makes it incapable of being controlled. (This is explicitly written into US federal laws for animal research, for example.) While we have certainly lowered the threshold for what animal suffering we will tolerate in a variety of animal uses, we do seem willing to accept some pain as inevitable in our social uses of animals. We still, after all, allow laboratory and zoo animals and farm animals to be housed in manners that patently violate their needs and natures and hurt them if there is no obvious available alternative.

As we remarked earlier, society is certainly more sensitive now to animal pain and suffering insofar as its concern has extended beyond cruelty. But insofar as much animal use seems to entail some pain and suffering, we limit our moral concern to 'manageable pain', rather than call the use occasioning pain 'unacceptable'. For example, we do not ban all animal research that causes pain; we ask that pain be controlled 'as far as possible', or that 'unnecessary pain be eliminated', and the yard-stick for necessity and possibility is human benefit and expediency. In other words, while we try to control animal pain and suffering consonant with our uses of these animals, we are unwilling to abandon most of our uses, and economic constraints limit our degree of moral concern. We will legally mandate control of pain in rodents used in research, but will not abandon all research where such control is impossible (e.g. pain research!) nor will we spend unlimited amounts to eliminate all suffering in research, such as that which is a consequence of keeping laboratory rodents in highly unnatural environments that violate their natures, but makes that research 'affordable'.

Even the most morally concerned, husbandry-based examples of animal use, such as western US extensive cattle ranching, where ranchers may spend more on treating an animal than the animal is worth, and where preserving a way of life looms larger as a motivation than profit does, must accept for practical reasons the infliction of pain on animals in management practices such as castration without anaesthesia and hot iron branding (or at least believe they must). Insofar as part of the way of life that ranchers are attempting to preserve requires making a living, ranchers cannot currently pursue their ideal of not inflicting pain, and accept as necessary the ultimate death of their charges (though few would voluntarily visit a slaughterhouse).

In other words, in most areas of animal use, the new ethic can only be imperfectly realised. So society does and will continue to focus on areas of animal use where pain and suffering are severe and obvious and where the path to their amelioration is clear, and to bracket the question of animal death as a moral issue. As most veterinarians will affirm, 'there are worse things that can happen to an animal than dying'. We have come to realise that there are many ways in which animals can suffer; we have become more sophisticated in recognising and controlling pain, but in the end, one moral imperative is clear: as much as possible, we must not allow animals to experience prolonged or intense pain and suffering at our hands.

The reasoning behind this moral insight is clear and ironically is augmented and potentiated by the arguments of those who would minimise our moral obligations to control animal pain. It was very common for the latter to affirm that animal pain is inherently trivial, since animals, lacking language and the conceptual tool box that language provides, live only in the now, in the moment. For humans, it is alleged, the real horror of pain comes from anticipating it, fearing and dreading it, dwelling upon one's past experiences of pain and extrapolating them to the future. If an animal's mental life is limited to a series of transient and ephemeral momentary 'nows', with no significant memory to rekindle past suffering, or anticipation or understanding to ignite trepidation about the future, then its pain is trivial as compared with a human's.

Suppose a person, the argument goes, say, a middle-aged man with a history of heart attacks, develops a sudden pain in the left arm. What makes such an experience terrible, it is said, is the memory of past experience that the sensation in question signals and the fear of what it betokens will happen–'Will I die?' 'Will I be incapacitated?' 'Is this the end?' For an animal, it is alleged, there is only the raw pain, without the attendant baggage. Thus, animal pain, it is alleged, is both momentary and of negligible moral significance compared to human pain.

There is, of course, an obvious rebuttal to this argument. It is plainly empirically false that animals live only in the moment and neither remember nor anticipate. A horse once shocked by an electric fence will avoid touching it; a dog once punished for stealing a canapé will grovel at a stern look or warning. And a cat will sit for hours anticipating the emergence of its prey.

But there is a far stronger moral point here. Suppose animals do in fact live only in the moment and humans do not. And suppose much of what makes a human's trip to the dentist so unpleasant is fear born of past experience and anticipation and paranoia: 'Suppose the dentist had a bad night? Suppose he is mad at me? Or mad at his wife and takes it out on me. Or suppose, as in the film *Marathon Man*, he is in fact Joseph Mengele', etc. Even if all this is true, it does not show that animal pain is more trivial then human. For on this hypothesis, animals lack something that mitigates pain for humans: they lack hope, understanding and power over their destiny. However much I fear the dentist, I know it will be over in twenty minutes. I know I can walk out. I know that the odds against the dentist being Mengele are 40 billion to 1. I can focus on the fact that in twenty minutes my toothache pain will be gone. Similarly with the arm pain: I know to call 911. I know to take a nitroglycerin tablet. I know that I will be at the hospital in five minutes and when I am told it is just indigestion, I hurt less.

An animal, however, has no such imaginative leeway if it is indeed stuck in the now. It cannot remember a time without pain, nor can it hope for such a time. Its entire universe is pain. Mentally it is the pain and nothing but the pain.

I seriously doubt for reasons suggested earlier that animals live *only* in the now. But I do believe that their limited cognitive abilities create a terrible *Erfahrungswelt* close to the model I described. Imagine a person who wakes up in a hospital room bandaged, intubated, and in terrible pain. Such a person can at the very least form some hypotheses — 'I've been in an accident', 'Someone will be here shortly', 'The pain will wear off', 'I'll call for help'. An animal waking up in such circumstances understands nothing, can formulate no hypothetical reassurances and has no strategy to make the hurt go away.

Common sense recognises the centrality of uncontrolled pain in an animal's life. Even hard core rednecks will more often than not stop their cars to 'put an injured animal out of its misery' if they have the means to do so; many hunters will go to extraordinary and arduous lengths to track a wounded animal to stop its pain. While we may argue endlessly about the morality of voluntary euthanasia for humans, few people will defend a person who keeps a suffering pet alive for their own needs. Indeed, in Sweden, animal oncology is not taught or practiced in veterinary school: the suffering occasioned is seen as far worse than the foreshortened life.

In sum, I would argue that unmitigated pain is the greatest evil for an animal, and that the most fundamental right flowing from *any* animal's *telos* is the right to have its pain alleviated or terminated. A dog in major and unmitigated pain is not a dog — its *telos* is ablated. And while we clearly cannot police a creation rife with suffering, we are certainly morally obliged to control whatever pain emerges from our use of animals for human benefit. Unfortunately, as we have discussed, while this moral obligation is as prominent in the social mind as it has ever been in the history of civilisation, we are far from realising it fully in most of our animal uses, for utilitarian and economic reasons.

The role of companion animals in society

There is, however, one area of animal use in society where our emerging ethic for animal treatment is fully realisable, even given the fact that we are unwilling to relinquish the benefits of that use. This is the area of companion animal use, wherein the tragic conflict between moral concern for animals and their benefit to humans does not arise. For companion animals are kept for basically one purpose — to give and receive love! And, unlike the situation with laboratory animals or food animals or zoo animals, there is nothing intrinsic in the companion relationship that requires hurting or killing animals. Quite the opposite in fact; if one loves something and is loved by it, hurting it or letting it suffer flies directly in the face of the logic of such a relationship!

The extent to which animals — primarily dogs and cats — fill the role of givers and receivers of love in our society is extraordinary and continues to grow. The overwhelming majority of pet owners in the United States are at least willing to affirm that their animals are members of the family — close to 99%, in fact. Every one of us knows of sane, affluent professional couples or singles who lavish enormous amounts of time and money on their pets as apparent child substitutes. Every divorce lawyer can tell stories of otherwise amicable divorce negotiations breaking down over the issue of custody of the dog or cat.

The role of such animals in giving and getting love is especially manifest in urban contexts. In a place like New York City, loneliness is an epidemic disease. One can live next door to a neighbour for twenty years and never exchange a greeting; that is in fact the norm. When one enters an elevator in an apartment house or public building, one automatically moves as far away from everyone else as possible, and develops a great interest in studying the ceiling. As much as possible, one avoids making eye contact with others; certainly one does not initiate conversations, especially with members of the opposite sex. One grows suspicious of everyone, and it is extremely difficult to make friends or even casual conversation. If one is single, divorced, widowed, new to the City, shy, lonely, or afraid, an animal, whether dog or cat, becomes a wonderful emotional resource. (The novels of Kinky Friedman beautifully illustrate the extent to which even an urbane, sophisticated, socially adroit New Yorker can bond with an animal.)

Not only does an animal provide companionship, it facilitates human companionship. The only strangers New Yorkers will freely address are those walking dogs or babies. People who know each other only as 'Fifi's master' or 'Brutus' person' developed an extraordinary sense of responsibility for one another in New York's dog-walking subculture, with the dogs serving as a social lubricant. A dog may be the only excuse one allows oneself for exercising, or the only way of instilling in a person a sense of security amid rampant fear. When I moved out of my New York apartment to live in Colorado, an ancient lady hugged my guard-trained Great Dane and affirmed, through tears, 'I'll never feel safe again'. With most marriages ending in divorce, an animal may well be the only solid and permanent source of unqualified affection or support to a child or even to an adult. And to the elderly, a pet may be nothing less than a reason to get up in the morning, to go out, to keep on living.

There is a relevant point in moral theory often forgotten and worth mentioning here. In our human relationships, we have moral obligations to all other humans. Even if I don't know you, I am obliged not to lie to you or assault you, or cheat you. But we have special obligations to those closest to us, for whom we are responsible. What would we think of a person who raised money for children starving in India and yet ignored the nutritional needs of his own children? For that matter, people would rightly think me blameworthy if I made charitable contributions to the United Way in a community 2000 miles away, while contributing nothing in my home town.

The same logic holds true of our moral obligation to animals. When we domesticated animals, and made them dependent on us for basic necessities of life, we incurred a moral obligation to meet their needs; that is one reason people find our treatment of farm animals in confinement agriculture so shocking. And this special obligation is *a fortiori* true of our interaction with companion animals, who not only rely wholly on us, but with whom we have personal relationships and to whom we have personal obligations. We may understandably forget our moral obligations to the pig we eat and have never met; but to forget your obligation to the 15-year-old dog who has loved you and helped raise you since you were a child is unforgivable. And, as we have argued, there is no more egregious and blameworthy form of neglect to an animal companion than to allow them to suffer pain that can be alleviated.

It is interesting to speculate how most pet owners would respond if faced by a choice of pressing a button and alleviating the cancer pain of their pets or pressing a second button and alleviating the equally severe pain of a stranger in Central Asia. If the choice were secret, I have little doubt that people would unhesitatingly choose surcease of pain for their pets, with little hesitation. As a matter of fact, people do *de facto* regularly choose the well-being of their own pets over that of alleviating human suffering — even child–suffering — *all the time.* How many of us would stop feeding our pets and dedicate the money to the relief of starving children? We answer that question daily in the negative!

The obvious question which initially arises is this: If I am correct, then why is there so little pain control in fact dispensed in companion animal practice? First of all, even the use of analgesia is relatively rare: Lloyd Davis has remarked that veterinarians regularly dispense antibiotics without documenting infection, yet withhold analgesia because they are not absolutely sure that pain is present, though unnecessary antibiotics do more harm than unnecessary analgesics. But indeed, until very recently, veterinary use of anesthesia was questionable, with many veterinarians using ketamine alone for cat spays, despite the total failure of ketamine to provide visceral pain control. We will return to this point.

Pain control and veterinary medicine

Few of us ignore animal pain willfully and knowingly. We in fact know little of animal pain because we know little of animals. Thus we may think of signs of pain from arthritis as a natural consequence of 'old age' rather than as a treatable problem and not treat it. We are only beginning to realise that at least part of the blame for loss of strength and fitness accompanying human ageing is our expectation and acceptance of it as inevitable! We may assume that our veterinarian is acutely conscious of pain of all sorts and is doing everything to treat it. Unfortunately, assuming this about veterinarians is as erroneous as assuming that our physicians are focussed in a major way on human pain, suffering, and quality of life rather than on effecting cures. For, in fact, throughout most of the twentieth century, veterinarians have been ill-prepared, by education and ideology, to manage animal pain in the same way that pain control has not historically been a priority for human physicians.

There are a variety of reasons that felt pain has been ignored in scientific medicine, human and veterinary, and it is worth briefly calling them to mind [6,7]. In the first place, all of science from Newton onwards, but primarily in the twentieth century, has laboured under an extremely positivistic ideology believed to demarcate science from speculation. This set of unexamined presuppositions assumes that science can deal only with what can be observed or tested and that all non-empirically verifiable notions should be removed from scientific discourse. To some extent, of course, this approach was laudable: it removed from physics suspect notions like absolute space and time and ether, and from biology empirically empty notions like life force and entelechy in the sense used by Driesch and others. Unfortunately, zealous prosecution of this idea threw out baby with bath water when it was declared that science had no place for value judgments (and *a fortiori* ethical judgements) or for talk of subjective experiences such as thoughts, feelings and pain, as denied by behaviourism, or for philosophical assertions.

This is bad philosophy. Science certainly makes value judgment when it affirms the epistemic superiority of experiment over anecdote, or the legitimacy of hurting or killing animals to make scientific progress. Science certainly presupposes — indeed founds itself upon — subjective experience when it affirms that only empirical judgments are scientifically admissible, for empirical judgments are founded on some scientist's observations, that is, they are ultimately subjective experiences. And science makes significant philosophical commitments when it goes from a scientist's first person reports to assuming an intersubjective external world existing independently of all subjects.

This bad philosophy has made for bad science and bad medicine. In its desire to eschew the unscientific, human medicine has largely ignored felt pain, and concentrated on 'cure' not 'care'. The most dramatic and egregious example of this historically is probably the failure to control cancer pain in 80% of human cancer patients even though 90% of such pain is controllable [8]. Equally horrifying is the fact that neonatal surgeons regularly performed open heart surgery on neonates using paralytic drugs until the late 1980s, and still perform a variety of procedures from colonoscopies and setting broken limbs to bone marrow aspiration using non-anaesthetic, non-analgesic amnesiacs such as short-acting benzodiazepines (Valium, Versed or Dormicum).

Another mischievous but little known component of scientific ideology is the current definition of pain accepted by the International

Society for the Study of Pain, which definition explicitly affirms that only beings with language are to be thought of as capable of feeling pain [9]. This Cartesian definition of course has major implications for animals as well as for young humans, and unfortunately, actual use of anaesthesia and analgesia in human medicine still follows this ideology.

Veterinary medicine of course followed human 'scientific' medicine's lead in historical agnosticism about animal pain, and the failure to consider animal pain was augmented by reasons unique to veterinary medicine. Until the late 1960s, veterinary medicine was overwhelmingly ancillary to agriculture, and the veterinarian's task was strictly dictated by the economic value of the animal, with the control of felt pain not of concern to producers and thus not expected of veterinary medicine. This is epitomized in Merillat's 1905 veterinary surgery textbook in which he laments the almost total disregard of anaesthesia in veterinary practice, with the episodic exception of the canine practitioner whose clients presumably valued their animals enough in non-economic terms to demand anesthesia [10].

As late as 1973, the first textbook of veterinary anesthesia published in the us, by Lumb and Jones, does not list the control of felt pain as a reason for using anaesthesia. Many veterinarians over 40 or 50 years of age still use the phrase 'chemical restraint' as synonymous with 'anaesthesia'; some were trained in the 1960s to castrate horses using curariform (paralytic) drugs like succinylcholine which not only do not mask or diminish felt pain, but probably intensify it by the fear they create. Others erroneously talk of anesthesia as 'sedation', though again most sedatives neither mask nor diminish pain.

Veterinary medicine had its own set of still-invoked rationalisations and ideological dogmas to vindicate not paying attention to pain control that one can still encounter today. One hears that anaesthesia is 'more stressful than the surgical procedure performed without anesthesia'. Post-surgical analgesics are not needed because animals will 'eat immediately after surgery'. Analgesics are not to be used because without the pain, the animal will inexorably re-injure the damaged body part. Post-surgical howling and whining are not signs of pain, they are 'after-effects of anaesthesia'. Anatomical differences, such as the presence of an anatomical mesenteric sling, vitiate the need for pain control after abdominal surgery in the dog. Animals do not need post-surgical analgesia because we can watch them behave normally after surgery. Young animals feel less pain that older ones, and thus do not need surgical anaesthesia for procedures like tail docking or castration, performed with 'bruticaine'. And so on.

There are, of course, answers to all of these shibboleths. I have attempted to provide such responses in my own writings [7,8], as have pioneering veterinarians such as Drs. Bernie Hansen and David Morton.

Equally important, it is now definitively known that uncontrolled pain is not only morally problematic when allowed to persist in animals, it is biologically deleterious. Unmitigated pain is biologically active as a major biological stressor, and affects numerous aspects of physical health, from wound-healing to resistance to infectious disease. One remarkable study showed that when pain in rats with cancer was controlled with analgesia *versus* not controlled, the rats given analgesia developed 80% fewer metastatic lesions [11]. The conclusion is inescapable: uncontrolled pain damages health and well-being, and can even, if pain is severe enough, engender mortality.

Unfortunately, most veterinarians know little about pain control, in particular about post-surgical analgesia. In the 1980s, as it became clear to those concerned about proper treatment of laboratory animals that there was little use of, knowledge of, or literature on laboratory animal analgesia, it became simultaneously clear that this was equally true in veterinary practice. Well into the 1990s and even today, it is clear that veterinarian knowledge of and training in use of analgesics is woefully inadequate, and that what is known by practitioners is typically not acquired in veterinary school [1,2].

During the 1970s and the early 1980s, I was part of a group consisting mostly of veterinarians who were attempting to effect better treatment for laboratory animals in the US by way of writing federal legislation. Our legislation in fact was passed in 1985 and is the basis for the current Animal Care and Use Committee oversight system. One of our major concerns was increasing researcher use of analgesics and other modalities for pain control. Faced with the ideological scepticism about and denial of animal pain, discussed above, we attempted to cut the ideologically based Gordian knot by legislating that animals felt pain. This has been very effective in the research community, and both acknowledgment of felt pain and knowledge and use of pain control has increased precipitously and exponentially since the passage of these laws. We also hoped that such knowledge and use would 'trickle down' from academic veterinary clinicians and researchers to practitioners. To some extent this is occurring, but much of the old ideology is alive and well. Indeed, the executive director of one major state veterinary association force complained to me that he simply cannot understand why so many veterinary clinicians are still so antagonistic towards administering post-surgical pain control when clients want it for their animals, are willing, indeed glad, to pay for it, and it is cheap and easy money for practitioners. Ideology dies hard.

Aside from veterinarians missing out on an easy modality for augmenting their income, the sporadic use of painkillers in companion animals is morally unacceptable for the reasons we discussed earlier. In addition, failure to control pain distances both human patients and animal owners from scientific medical practitioners, human and veterinary. In my view, this has been a major factor spurring the rapid metastatic growth of alternative medicine in both fields. Alternative therapists at least appreciate the significance of pain and make sympathetic noises about it.

We are a society with little tolerance for discomfort of any sort: one only has to look at the astounding proliferation of over-the-counter and prescription remedies aimed at everything from baldness and haemorrhoids to back pain and soft erections. We will no longer tolerate those who extol the virtue of manly tolerance of suffering, nor patronise those who do nothing to alleviate it. And this is as true of our view of companion animals as it is for our children and ourselves.

A society that spends money on anxiolytic drugs for pets will not tolerate agnosticism about animal pain and reluctance to control it.

Pain management and education

How, then, do we bring veterinary medicine into accord with the emerging social ethic for companion animals? There is, in my view, only one answer – education. Admittedly, this is a cliché, but that does not make it false. And I would propose a very specific agenda for an educational *Blitzkrieg*.

One thrust must be directed towards clients. They must be taught to recognise known signs of pain, suffering, and discomfort in their companion animals. Secondly, they must be taught that their concern for animal pain is not silly, but perfectly legitimate ethically, even as clients have learned that grief for loss of pets is neither wimpish nor uncommon. Third, they must be taught to expect that their veterinarians be knowledgeable and morally concerned about animal pain.

On the veterinary side, education is also essential. Continuing education courses on pain identification, mechanisms, and control are essential. But this is only half the battle. Veterinarians, and especially the older practitioners, must be taught *good philosophy* to supplant the ideology they learned. Not only must they learn the philosophical basis for the legitimacy of talking about pain in animals, they must learn enough philosophy of science to see that what they learned in the past was bad philosophy and why it is bad philosophy. They must be made to understand that animal (and human) feelings like pain are not outside the ken of science. And they must be made to understand the general point that neither science nor medicine is value-free in general nor ethics-free in particular. They must be taught to understand the new ethic for animals and its application to companion animals so that they understand that client demand for pain-control is a non-negotiable, morally based demand.

Even more important, the same ideas must be inculcated into veterinary students. They must understand the historical and ideological reasons why some of their future employers are not interested in pain control, as well as how to deal with such veterinarians, so that the student's idealistic commitment to controlling pain, distress, and suffering is not blunted by crashing into the old ideology; and additional research demonstrating the value of pain control should be supported and disseminated.

Finally, the public in general should be made aware of progress in this area, particularly through television specials of the sort that highlight what we are learning about animal thought. Animal pain and its control is surely of like interest to great numbers of people, both because it is intrinsically interesting and because, in any case, as promoters of the new ethic we described, members of society have already committed to an interest in animal pain and its control.

There is no reason to believe that social intoxication with companion animals will wane, especially as we get older as a society. One of the most profound human needs is the need to be needed, and the need to care for others. Companion animals fill this role admirably, but our relationship with these animals is marred and blackened by our inability to understand their needs and natures, leading to totally preventable infliction of suffering on these animals, and also to the premature degradation and death of millions of these animals due to human inability to manage them. If we can require that people take driving courses before they are allowed to get cars, we can at least offer education in basic principles of husbandry of companion animals, covering nutrition, behaviour, training, ethics, etc. A major component of such education, be it mandatory as a necessary condition for acquiring a companion animal or elective in high school or college, should surely be familiarity with recognising and alleviating various modes of animal pain and suffering. Here, at least, is an animal issue where it is possible to orchestrate a solution which is win–win for all parties.

Selected bibliography

1 Gaskell G et al. Europe ambivalent on biotechnology. Nature 1997; 387:845 ff.

2 Singer P. Animal Liberation. Avon, New York 1991 (Originally published 1976).

3 Rollin B. Animal Rights and Human Morality. Prometheus, Buffalo, NY 1992 (Originally published 1981).

4 Regan T. The Case for Animal Rights. University of California Press, Berkeley 1985.

5 Sapontzis S. Morals, Reason, and Animals. Temple University Press, Philadelphia 1987.

6 Rollin B. The Unheeded Cry: Animal Consciousness, Animal Pain and Science. Iowa State University Press, Ames, Iowa 1988. (Originally published Oxford University Press, 1989)

7 Rollin B. Pain and ideology in human and veterinary medicine. Seminars in Veterinary Medicine and Surgery (Small Animals) 1997; 12(no.2):56-60.

8 Ferrell BR, Rhiner M. High-tech Comfort: Ethical issues in cancer pain management for the 1990s. Journal of Clinical Ethics 1991; 2:108-15.

9 Rollin B. Some conceptual and ethical concerns about current views of pain. Pain Forum 1999;8(2):78-83.

10 Merillat LA. Principles of Veterinary Surgery. Alexander Eger, Chicago 1999.

11 Page GG, Ben-Eliyahu S, Yirmiyah R, Lebeskind J. Morphine attenuates surgery-induced enhancement of metastatic colonization in rats. Pain 1993;54:21-8.

12 Dohoo SE, Dohoo IR. Postoperative use of analgesics in dogs and cats by Canadian veterinarians. Can Vet J 1996;36:546-51.

13 Dohoo SE, Dohoo IR. Factors influencing the postoperative use of analgesics in dogs and cats by Canadian veterinarians. Can Vet J 1996; 37:552-6.

3

CHANGING ROLES OF ANIMALS IN SOCIETY

Nienke Endenburg, PhD,
Faculty of Veterinary Medicine,
Utrecht University, Utrecht, The Netherlands

Introduction

People have kept pets since prehistoric times [1]. No society and no culture has lived without animals [2]. Man hunted animals [3,4] and later on domesticated them [5-7]. After domestication, animals were not only used for functional purposes but also played an important role as companions. The existence of pet-keeping among so-called 'primitive' people poses a problem for those who choose to believe that such behaviour is the product of Western wealth, decadence and bourgeois sentimentality. They could hardly be described as either wealthy or decadent [1].

As can be seen in ancient paintings, almost every culture developed its own dog breed. In the Far East, this was the Pekinese, a companion animal that became a very important member of the family. In the ancient world, people held the belief that animals, because they were rational, knew the difference between right and wrong, and could be held accountable for their acts [8]. In the Middle Ages, people continued to believe in the accountability of animals for their misdeeds [9]: animals were personified and were entitled to the same legal protection as humans [10].

From the Middle Ages to the beginning of the nineteenth century, people of the Western world were involved in agricultural improvement and exploitation. It was seen as a moral obligation. In 1630 the French philosopher, René Descartes proposed that animals were merely complex machines, like clocks, capable of a variety of automatic functions, but totally incapable of conscious thought, or even sensation. Only humans possessed minds and rational souls;

animals were merely mindless and soulless automata. This attitude made it possible to treat animals as beings without pain. So people enjoyed seeing cruel games like bull-baiting, bear-baiting, cock-fighting and dog-fighting.

After the Second World War there was a change in pet keeping in the Western world. There are a number of aspects that were responsible for this.

– *The increasing prosperity made it possible for many people to own companion animals (in Western society). In many other cultures/countries not as prosperous as most western countries, animals are also kept solely for companionship, but not in such large numbers [1]. The increasing welfare of western society made it possible to spend money on animals that were kept only for company, and that were and sometimes still are seen as luxury.*

– *Increasing mobility and the resulting loosening of ties with the extended family [11]. In earlier days it was normal for members of the family to interact with each other. They supported each other and satisfied each other's social needs. Nowadays this is often no longer the case. The two-generation family is what remains.*

– *The family lost many of its economic and legal socialisation functions. The family as a source of emotional satisfaction has become more important during the last few decades. From Maslow's scheme [12] it can easily be deduced that when primary and secondary needs are fulfilled, emotional needs become important. More will be demanded of the quality of relationships, which will make disappointments inevitable. Those disappointments concern human relationships [13]. In other words, the pressure on the two-generation family for the satisfaction of emotional needs has become very strong. Companion animals could be a way to lower this pressure.*

– *People have lost contact with nature [14]. The interaction with companion animals gives people a way to interact with nature and restore this lost contact. This can also influence their health.*

It might well be that human beings in western society felt an increasing need to satisfy their emotional needs, which was not always possible by means of other human beings, so that the function of the animal has changed and the companionship role has become more important. This might be the reason that more companion animals are kept and that their impact on the life of human beings has gained more attention. Also the affection, touch, and comfort provided by the contact with other beings are important and give people the chance to interact with nature [14]. In this respect, animals could fulfil a function as well.

This change in keeping animals also resulted in the creation of a new term — companion animals. These animals fulfil a recreational function. Companion animals fulfil the needs of people to have these animals around them. These animals may be dogs and cats, but nowadays people also keep sheep, horses and pigs as companion animals. The emotional value of these animals is higher than their economic value. They are individuals who have their own names and their owners will develop an emotional bond with them. In this chapter, the term companion animal will be used only for dogs, cats, rabbits, rodents, fish, birds, and horses.

Influence of companion animals on humans

Contact with companion animals can enhance the quality of life of their human partners. Indicators of human well-being are found in the following categories: psychological, social, behavioural, and physiological. Well being or quality of life can be, as has been shown by (recent) research, considerably improved when people have companion animals. Below, the aspects of human well-being and the influence pets have on them, will be discussed.

Psychological well-being

The main theme of research here is the study into loneliness defined as subjective feelings of loneliness or social isolation. For instance, in one study it was found that women college students living alone were lonelier than those who were living with a pet [15]. In several other studies, however, there was no influence of pets on loneliness [16].

Behavioural well-being

Allen and co-workers [17] introduced a pet- or best friend support, as compared with a control condition. They examined the effects of pets or friends present on the performance of arithmetic calculations. This behavioural indicator of well-being showed a clear advantage in favour of pet presence over that of a friend.

Physical well-being

Physical well-being, in connection to owning one or more pets, is most frequently quantified by cardiovascular responses and (minor) health complaints. Studies indicate that a dog may reduce cardiovascular stress responses in man. Friedmann et al. [18] showed that the presence of a friendly dog during reading and resting reduced systolic and diastolic blood pressure in children. Grossberg et al. [19] showed that when students had a conversation with a researcher or read aloud, their blood pressure increased more than when they talked to, and petted, an unfamiliar dog. Wilson [20] showed that blood pressure during petting a dog was significantly lower than during a baseline period. A parallel effect was demonstrated by reading quietly.

Anderson et al. [21] showed that owning a companion animal might also have a long lasting effect; pet owners had significant lower systolic blood pressures, triglyceride and cholesterol levels than people who did not own pets. These authors suggested that pet ownership might moderate cardiovascular risk factors, and therefore prevent cardiovascular disease. This was in accordance with an American study in which pet owners were found to be more likely to be alive one year after hospital admission for coronary problems than people who did not own a pet [22]. This effect was not related to the increased exercise levels of dog owners or to the severity of the illness. Although many studies indicate that companion animals may have a stress reducing effect, not all reported studies support this [23]. Grossberg et al. [24] for example, did not find significant differences in blood pressure or heart rate between students performing arithmetic tasks with or without the presence of their own dog.

Social well-being

The main research theme in this area is social support. The concept of social support comes from the research and development done in human social support theory and reported in literature. It relates to the social support given by other people. Support may be given in different forms such as money, shelter or transportation. But the support may also be emotional, with expressions of sympathy and esteem for, and confidence in, the recipient. Research in the human–animal bond concerns mainly the emotional support. Companion animals can give emotional support in a direct and indirect way: in a direct way because owners can feel more confident and will not feel alone when they have a pet. Indirectly, people with pets develop more social contacts with other human beings than they would have without pets. Pets thereby function as catalysts in human contacts.

The conclusion from the above-mentioned research is that the benefits of pets are evident in these fields. More research is needed because the 'quality-of-life' benefits of pet association are apparent only in certain situations and under certain circumstances. This research should be done with a consistent methodology, in order to elucidate when pet associations are beneficial.

The reasons people develop relationships with animals are various and reflect the human's personality and attitudes. The relationship that develops with companion animals is comparable to that which we develop with human companions and can vary in intensity and form in a similar way. The differences in types of relationship may be due to variations in the behavioural characteristics of either the humans or the animals involved. In addition, the more similar the social organisation and communication systems of the two species, the more likely it is that each will recognise signals from the other and be able to respond appropriately. This similarity, especially with regard to communication and sensory systems, tends to be greater between the 'higher' vertebrates and humans and therefore we are more likely to have a closer relationship with a dog or a cat than we are with fish or reptiles [25].

Most pet owners see their animal as a member of the family. Owners celebrate the birthday of the pet and very often they carry, next to the photos of their human family or loved one, pictures of their pets, in their purse. Sometimes owners even speak about their animals in terms of 'their child', and more and more people dress their pets as humans including perfume, nail polish and jewellery.

The aforementioned similarity can be held responsible for the fact that we anthropomorphise our cats and dogs, giving them humanlike characteristics and traits. Human emotions, thoughts, and behaviours are thus often attributed to animals despite the fact that little or no scientific evidence exists to support the presence of such characteristics. Owners have the feeling that their dog 'looked guilty' when he urinated inside or when he ran away from home. These omissions are held despite the fact that it is not clear whether or not animals can feel guilty. This is similar to the Middle Ages, when people believed in the accountability of animals for their misdeeds (see earlier). On the other hand, anthropomorphism may play an important role in the formation of the human-animal bond [26]. So we need to (and probably most owners do) anthropomorphise; we probably have no other opportunity to form a bond. If this is true, the question is how to prevent denying the needs of companion animals while anthropomorphising them. The denial of the needs of animals can easily happen as a consequence of attributing human emotions, thoughts and behaviours to animals. We need to balance between forming a bond with animals, knowing that we anthropomorphise them, and consider the animal as it is. Denial of the needs of animals can lead, for instance, to the development of behaviour problems or induce problems in the interaction between owner and animal. This ultimately can lead to the abandonment or the euthanasia of the animal, when owners cannot cope with the situation any longer.

Thus, to experience any feeling of interaction, people must be able to interpret the 'language' and the behaviour of animals [27]. Furthermore, the more 'sensitive' a companion animal is to an owner's signal, the greater the attachment that can develop between person and animal. The idea of 'sensitive' responsiveness frequently appears in the literature relating to human attachment relations [28–30]. It refers to the degree in which an 'attaching' figure notices the signals of the child, interprets them correctly, and is ready and prepared to react affectively to evoke a feeling of trust and accessibility [28]. Bowlby is generally considered to be the founder of attachment theory. He defined attachment as 'a lasting emotional tie between people such that the individual strives to maintain closeness to the object of attachment and acts to ensure the relationship continues' [31].

The strong attachments that people form with their animals are due to several factors including anthropomorphised behaviours, companion rather than utilitarian roles, easily misinterpreted communication signals, and living conditions (usually freedom from enclosures such as cages or pens, which allow animals to share daily routines and leisure-time activities with humans [26]. Pets who are viewed as sources of emotional and social support and are treated as family members are likely to elicit strong feelings of attachment from their owners [26].

Cognitive dissonance

So far, the positive effects of the human-animal bond have been described. The life span of pets is, however, shorter than that of owners. Pets will die or become ill, and most owners will survive their animals. The fact that (even young) animals can be in great pain sometimes makes it necessary to consider euthanasia. For owners this can be a very difficult decision, especially when the animal's condition deteriorates slowly. This because the owner is now confronted with two contradictory cognitions. Cognition includes thoughts, attitudes, beliefs, and also behaviours of which a person is aware. Two relevant cognitions may exist either in a state of consonance or in a state of dissonance. When dissonance occurs, the two elements do not fit with each other: the one element implies the opposite of the other (I am a responsible pet owner and I do not want my animal to be in pain; I will miss my pet terribly when it is no longer alive). This is called the cognitive dissonance [32]. Cognitive dissonance is said to exist when a person has two cognitions that contradict each other. Dissonance, the theory suggests, is an uncomfortable state from which the individual will try to escape by altering some of his or her cognitions or behaviour. Most owners have their limits. They will tell themselves and others for instance that if the dog can walk around the block, he is feeling fine. But when he cannot any longer walk around the block, they then have two cognitions that contradict each other. The solution to this problem can be that owners say the dog is still all right when he can walk half the block. But most often it is very difficult to make an estimation how much pain animals have.

Pain behaviour is not always observed by the owners, because we tend to look at animals the same way as we look at our fellow human beings. Human beings are mostly able to tell or to vocalise when in pain; most animals are not able to do this. Animals show that they have pain in a different way. Owners observe their animals, and are sometimes able to see or notice that their animal is behaving in a different way. They can notice that there is a change in routine — for instance the animal does not play anymore. At the weekends, owners generally have more time to observe the animal, and problems become suddenly clear, so a veterinarian is needed then.

Well-being of animals

As stated before, owners or caretakers of animals often see their pets as a part of the family. These people will worry about the animal when they feel that the well-being of the pet is negatively affected. This is especially the case when the animal is in pain.

But what is the actual meaning of the well-being of animals? From the literature, there does not seem to be an unambiguous view. Some scientists assume that the animal is afflicted in its well-being when their possibility to survive and to reproduce is decreased [33]. Broom [34] holds the same opinion but remarks that a heavily wounded animal is also afflicted in its well-being when it is sleeping or under anaesthesia. In his view, even in the absence of physical problems, but when the animal is frightened, scared, frustrated or bored, its well-being is decreased. Other researchers [35–38] showed that feelings of animals are the most important concerning well-being. They assume that well-being is decreased when it feels mentally unpleasant. These researchers imply that an unpleasant mental state is found in an animal that is frightened, anxious, frustrated or bored. For these scientists, an animal with a tumour that is not causing physical and mental problems, there is no decreased well-being. When looking into the topic of well-being, it is obvious that there are several definitions.

A decreased well-being of the animal may result in the well-being of humans being decreased, because of the bond between the human family members and the animal. People worry about the animal, how it is to be treated best, and whether or not it will survive.

When the animal is in pain it can be stated that the well-being of the animal is decreased. When the owner decides to have the animal euthanised, the bond between the animal and the owner is broken. In fact, the death of a companion animal may be one of the most significant losses that people, adults and children alike, experience in their lives [39,40]. The fact that the animal is in pain or has to be euthanised very often has a considerable influence on the owner. A grieving process quite often will follow the euthanasia. Grief is the natural and spontaneous response to loss, and is essential for healing the emotional wounds. Grief when a human family member dies is associated with a variety of mental en physical health consequences [41]. Whether or not the same effects will happen when a pet dies is the topic of presently ongoing research. Experiences of bereaved pet owners suggest this to be so.

References

1   Serpell JA. In the Company of Animals: A study of human-animal relationships. Basil Blackwell, Oxford 1986.
2   Noske B. Huilen met de wolven. Een interdisciplinaire benadering van de mens-dier relatie. van Gennep, Amsterdam 1988.
3   Lee R, DeVore J. Man the Hunter. Aldine, Chicago 1968.
4   Fox M. Relationships between the human and non-human animals. In: Fogle B (Ed). Interrelations between People and Pets. Charles C. Thomas, Springfield, Illinois 1981.

5   Canby TY. The search for the first Americans. Natl. Geographic 1979;156(3):348.

6   Davis SJM, Valla FR. Evidence for domestication of the dog 12,000 years ago in the Natufian of Israel. Nature 1978;276:608-10.

7   Messent PR. Behavioural patterns of companion animals - their significance in pet/owner bonding. Proceedings of meeting Group study of human companion animal bond. Dundee, 1979.

8   Levinson BM. Pet-oriented Child Psychotherapy. Charles C.Thomas, Springfield, Illinois 1969.

9   Veper GM. Les proces des animaux au moyen age. Cour d'appel de Chambery, Chambery 1954.

10 Hyde WW. The prosecution and punishment of animals and lifeless things in the middle ages and modern times. University of Pennsylvania Law Review 1915/16;64:696-730.

11 Arkow P. Dynamic Relationships in Practice: Animals in the helping profession. The Latham Foundation, Alameda 1984.

12 Maslow AH. Motivation and Personality. Harper and Row, New York 1954.

13 Tromp G. Het dier als vriend. In: Visser MBH, Grommers FJ (Eds). Dier en Ding, Objectivering van dieren. Pudoc, Wageningen 1988:73-85.

14 Katcher AH. Interactions between people and their pets: form and function. In: Fogle B (Ed). Interrelations between People and Pets. Charles C. Thomas, Springfield, Illinois 1981:41-67.

15 Zasloff RL, Kidd AH. Loneliness and pet ownership among single women. Psychological Reports 1994;75:747-52.

16 Garrity THF, Stallones L. Effects of pet contact on human well-being. In: Wilson CC, Turner DC (Eds). Companion Animals in Human Health, Sage, California 1998:3-22.

17 Allen KM, Blascovich J, Tomaka J, Kelsey RM. Presence of human friends and pet dogs as moderators of autonomic responses to stress in women. Journal of Personality and Social Psychology 1991;61:582-9.

18 Friedmann E, Katcher AH, Thomas SA, Lynch JJ, Messent PR. Social interaction and blood pressure: The influence of animal companions. Journal of Nervous and Mental Disease 1983; 171:461-5.

19 Grossberg JM, Alf EF. Interaction with pet dogs: Effects on human cardiovascular response. Journal of the Delta Society 1985;2:20-7.

20 Wilson CC. Physiological responses of college students to a pet. Journal of Nervous and Mental Disease 1975:606-12.

21 Anderson WP, Reid CM, Jennings GL. Pet ownership and risk factors for cardiovascular disease. The Medical Journal of Australia 1992;157:298-301.

22 Friedmann E, Katcher AH, Lynch JJ, Thomas SA. Animal companions and one-year survival of patients after discharge from a coronary care unit. Public Health Reports 1980;95:307-12.

23 Straatman I, Hanson EKS, Endenburg N, Mol JA. The influence of a dog on male students during a stressor. Anthrozoös 1997;10(4):191-7.

24 Grossberg JM, Alf EF, Vormbrock JK. Does pet dog presence reduce human cardiovascular responses to stress? Anthrozoös 1988;2:38-44.

25 Robinson I. Associations between man and animals. In: Robinson I (Ed). The Waltham Book of Human-Animal Interaction: Benefits and responsibilities of pet ownership. Pergamon, Oxford 1995:1-6.

26 Lagoni L, Butler C, Hetts S. The Human-Animal Bond and Grief. W.B.Saunders Company, Philadelphia 1994.

27 Endenburg N. The attachment of people to companion animals. Anthrozoos 1995;VIII(2):83-9.

28 Ainsworth MD, Blehar MC, Waters E, Wall S. Patterns of attachment. A psychological study of the strange situation. Erlhaum, Hillsdale, NY 1978.

29 IJzendoorn MH van, Lambermon MWE. Transgenerationele overdracht van gehechtheid en verbreding van het opvoedingsmilieu. In: Goudena, PP, Groenendaal HJ, Swets-Gronert FA. Kind in Het Geding. Acco, Amersfoort 1988.

30 Tuyl C van. Sensitieve responsiviteit; een conceptuele analyse. ISOR, Utrecht 1993.

31 Bowlby J. Attachment and Loss. Vol. 1: Attachment. Hogarth Press, London 1969.

32 Festinger L. A Theory of Cognitive Dissonance. Standford University Press, Stanford, CA 1957.

33 Barnett JL, Hemsworth PH. The validity of physiological and behavioural measures of animal welfare. Applied Animal Behaviour Science 1990;18:133-42.

34 Broom DM. Assessing welfare and suffering. Behavioural Processes 1991;25:117-23.

35 Dawkins M. Animal Suffering: The science of animal welfare. Chapman and Hall, London 1980.

36 Dawkins M. From an animal's point of view: motivation, fitness and animal welfare. Behavioural and Brain Sciences 1990;13:1-61.

37 Duncan IJH, Petherick JC. Cognition: the implications for animal welfare. Applied Animal Behaviour Science 1989;24:81.

38 Sandoe P, Simonsen HP. Assessing animal welfare: where does science end and philosophy begin? Animal welfare 1992;1:257-67.

39 Gage G, Holcomb R. Couples' perceptions of the stressfulness of the death of the family pet. Family Relations 1991;40:103-5.

40 Hart LA, Hart BL, Mader B. Humane euthanasia and companion animal death: Caring for the animal, the client, and the veterinarian. Special commentary. Journal of the American Veterinary Medical Association 1990;197:1292-9.

41 Stroebe MS, Stroebe W, Hansson RO. Bereavement research and theory: An introduction to the Handbook. In: Stroebe MS, Stroebe W, Hansson RO (Eds); Handbook of Bereavement, Cambridge University Press, Cambridge 1993.

4

RECOGNITION OF PAIN BEHAVIOUR IN ANIMALS

Elizabeth M. Hardie, DVM, PhD, DipACVS,
College of Veterinary Medicine,
North Carolina State University, Raleigh, NC, USA

Introduction and doctrine of comparative biology

Veterinarians and animal caretakers use behavioural observations on a daily basis to assess the well-being of their charges. It therefore seems intuitive that recognition of pain ought to be easy. Unfortunately, it is not easy and is not always intuitive. Pain is an individual experience and how much of that experience translates into observable, measurable behaviour depends on a number of factors. Some of those variables include species, genetic line within the species, sex, weight of the animal, previous conditioning, social dominance of the animal, overall health of the animal and environmental conditions at the time of observation [1-6]. Animals cannot describe their pain; thus the biases of the observer enter into any method used to measure behaviour. Knowledge of the individual animal's normal behaviour, knowledge of species behaviour, observational skill and attitudes towards pain and pain behaviour all influence how an observer will judge or score an animal's pain.

The general consensus among investigators who use many methods to assess pain is that behavioural observation is a useful tool to distinguish between no pain and moderate to severe pain. When rigorous standardisation (single observer, use of videotapes, quantitative measurement) is applied, behavioural methods will distinguish between lesser pain levels and more severe pain levels.

The difficulties encountered in behavioural pain measurement have resulted in a doctrine that gives all animals the benefit of the doubt [7]. Animals are assumed to have nervous systems similar to adult humans. Any procedure or injury that is reported to be painful by verbal adult humans is considered to be painful in animals, even if they do not show overt behavioural evidence of pain. This doctrine is used by veterinarians and animal care committees as a guideline for supplying analgesic therapy. The guideline is a starting place only. It says nothing about how to assess if analgesic therapy is effective or how to address procedures and painful conditions that have no counterpart in humans.

Pain models

The simplest methods for using behaviour to assess pain involve observation of reflexes in response to an acute painful stimulus [8]. An electrical, thermal or mechanical stimulus is applied to a body part, usually the tail or limb, and the time to movement or withdrawal is measured. The advantages of these tests are that they are objective, easily measurable and distinguish between various analgesic interventions. The disadvantage is that reflexes are simply reflexes, not pain. Results of these tests may not mirror results in actual painful conditions.

The next level of complexity is to measure organised unlearned behaviours in response to a painful stimulus [6,8]. These tests require that the animal perceive the pain at a supra-spinal level and translate that perception into a response. An example is the hot plate test, in which a rodent is placed on an uncomfortably warm surface [6,9,10]. Three categories of behaviour are commonly seen on first exposure to the hot plate: sniffing responses, primary noxious evoked patterns (forepaw licking, hindpaw licking, stamping) and escape noxious evoked patterns (leaning posture, jumping off). Hind leg withdrawal and freezing in place are also seen, but do not cluster with any of the other behaviours. It appears that recording both the latency and the duration of the primary evoked noxious patterns tests the threshold for pain, while counting all behaviours more clearly characterises pain tolerance and analgesia. Learning is a problem with this model: the rodents quickly learn to lean and jump as soon as they are placed on the hot surface, confounding results. For example, the results of a morphine assay are different if a single animal is given several doses of morphine and repeatedly tested, rather than using many animals given different doses of morphine and tested only once.

The hot plate test measures the response to somatic pain. For visceral pain, a balloon is placed in the colon and inflated until a motor response such as head turning, abdominal contraction or foot shifting is observed [11,12]. The hot plate test and the colonic balloon tests are easily standardised and distinguish between analgesic interventions, but do not provide any data regarding the efficacy of drugs against the inflammatory component of pain.

Inflammatory pain can be measured by injecting an irritating substance (formalin, carragenin) into a footpad or joint and observing flinching, favouring the leg, licking of the leg, and lifting of the leg [8,13]. Objective counts of the number of licks, length of time of non-weight bearing on the affected limb, limb withdrawal time/vocalisation in response to a noxious stimulus, and locomotion over time within a designated space (open field test) are used to quantify the pain response. A more severe model, which mimics visceral inflammatory pain, relies on observation of the writhing response when irritating substances are injected into the peritoneum [8,14].

Observation of unlearned behaviour is also used to assess the response to more long lasting pain. Chronic neuropathic pain can be produced by complete or partial denervation of a limb, but models in which the behavioural endpoint is self-mutilation are considered inhumane [8,15]. More commonly, models are used which result in abnormal positions of the paw (lameness) and altered limb withdrawal in response to mechanical and thermal challenges.

Pain researchers may also use observation of learned behaviour [8]. For example, the animal is trained to perform some task, such as bar pressing or jumping over a barrier, to avoid a painful stimulus. The intensity at which this task is performed can be measured. In graded tests, the stimulus intensity is modified according to the number of times the task is performed. These tests allow investigators to measure pain thresholds and tolerances, but do not help the clinician trying to assess pain in untrained animals.

Table 1
Behaviours suggested by several authors [4,16-18] as being indicative of pain in animals.

Aspect of behaviour	General	Comments
Temperament	A change of temperament, either to aggressive or withdrawn. Aggression in response to forced movement of painful area.	Well socialised animals may display displacement activities during handling to avoid aggression directed towards a human handler.
Vocalisation	Vocalisation in response to palpation or movement of painful area.	Type of vocalisation unique to species. Increased anxiety may result in overall
Posture, Locomotion	Guarding of the painful area. Severe abdominal pain may result in hunched posture, falling and/or rolling.	Reluctance to move painful body part results in abnormal gait, stilted movements.
Facial expression	Exact changes species specific, generally dull eyes, 'staring into space', drooping ears. Grimace in some species.	Handler approach may elicit fear expression: dilated pupils, pinned back ears.
Grooming	Decreased normal grooming, unkept hair coat. Piloerection. Licking, kicking, biting or scratching painful area. Self-mutilation if pain is severe.	Reluctance to move or groom may cause soiling with faeces, urine.
Activity level	Restlessness or overall decrease in activity level.	Sleep patterns disturbed, often increased activity when sleep should be occurring.
Food and water consumption	Decreased.	

Table 2

Species specific acute pain behaviours suggested by several experts [4,16-18].

Species	Characteristic acute pain behaviours
Dog	Attention seeking, whining, whimpering, and howling common. Vocalisation often stops when animal is comforted. Rarely 'hides' painful body part. Hunched or 'prayer' posture with abdominal pain. Shivering, panting.
Cat	Vocalisation rare. Hissing or growling when approached or handled. Tendency to hide in enclosed space. Tendency to 'hide' painful body part, acting normal. Decreased activity, lack of grooming, hunched posture, dissociation from environment with severe pain. Aggression if approached or painful area is moved.
Horse	Colic pain signs include periods of restlessness, standing with head lowered, interrupted eating, anxious expression with dilated pupils and glassy eyes, flaring of the nostrils, sweating, rigid posture, repeated standing up and lying down, head turning or kicking towards the abdomen, and rolling. Reluctance to be handled. Less severe pain usually results in dull expression, dissociation from surroundings, teeth grinding, poor appetite.
Cow, Sheep, Goats	Dull expression, dissociation from surroundings, reluctance to move, rigid body stance. Colic signs similar to horses, but less severe. Teeth grinding, grunting. Handling may provoke aggression. Vocalisation rare, except in goats.
Pig	Overt pain behaviour rare. Lack of normal social behaviour and vocalisation may indicate pain. Vocalisation in response to handling may be more pronounced. Changes in gait, reluctance to move, hiding in bedding.
Laboratory rodents	Overt pain behaviour rare. Decreased food consumption, decreased locomotion after major surgery. Severe abdominal pain causes writhing. Squeals audible by humans produced in response to palpation of painful area.

Acute pain states

What does an animal in acute pain look like? There have been numerous attempts to answer this question. The collective wisdom of experienced observers has been used to draw up a list of possible behaviours for each species (Tables 1,2).

More objectively, animals undergoing a painful procedure have been compared to sham controls or to themselves before the procedure (Table 3).

What becomes apparent is that it requires an extremely painful experience for the most obvious behaviours to occur. Examples would be vocalisation, rolling, falling down and aggression during the palpation of the painful site. These behaviours are infrequent and large group numbers are needed to demonstrate significant differences between the painful animals and controls. Pain in the moderate range produces changes in body position and posture, eating, sleep patterns, grooming patterns and locomotion. These behavioural changes may be difficult to perceive during short-term behavioural observations and can be associated with sedation, stress or illness as well as pain.

Another method of establishing whether or not a behaviour is associated with acute pain is to take a group of animals undergoing a painful procedure, give some of the animals a known analgesic drug and some a placebo drug, and then observe behavioural differences between the groups (Table 4).

Most of these studies have used global pain scores to judge pain, rather than listing individual behaviours. Observers can usually judge if an animal has received an analgesic, but multi-point scales often have to be collapsed into two point scales (comfortable/uncomfortable, needs intervention analgesia/does not need intervention analgesia) in order to demonstrate significant differences between treated and untreated groups [30-32]. Subtle differences between various doses of analgesics appear to be best demonstrated using summed quantitative measurements such as locomotor activity or body weight changes [6,33].

Table 3
Examples of acute pain behaviours documented by comparison with non-painful controls.

Reference number	Subjects group size	Painful Procedure	Controls	Behaviour change
19	Dairy cows N=8	Hot branding, freeze branding	Sham branding	No vocalisations in any groups. Hot branded cows kicked more than other groups.
20	Beef calves N=8	Hot branding, freeze branding	Sham branding	No difference in vocalisation between groups. Hot branded calves jumped further than other groups.
21	Feedlot steers N=100	Hot branding, freeze branding	Sham branding	Hot branded cows had greater tail-flick, kick, fall in chute, and vocalisation frequencies than other groups. Freeze branded cows had greater tail-flick frequency than controls.
22	Lambs N=6	Tail docking and castration using 2 sizes of rubber rings, crushing, or both	Similar handling and sampling, no surgery	The frequency of foot stamping, restlessness and tail flicking was higher in the ring groups than other groups. The time spent in abnormal postures (lateral lying, sternal lying, dog sitting, statue standing) was higher in ring groups than other procedure groups and all procedure groups were higher than controls. Rolling and kicking were seen only in the ring groups.
23	Mice N=6	Intraperitoneal injection, 3 doses of Freund's incomplete adjuvent	Saline injected controls	Dose dependent changes in body weight and nocturnal locomotor activity. No changes in open field test, clinical scoring. A few animals showed evidence of poor grooming.
24	Rats N=8	Laparotomy	Themselves, 4 sham controls	Disturbed circadian rhythms in locomotor activity for 2-5 days
25	Rats N=8-10	Nephrectomy, jugular catheter placement	Sham controls	Decreased locomotor activity, decreased food consumption, and decreased water consumption in surgery groups.
26	Horses N=13	Orthopaedic surgery	Themselves, pre-operatively	No significant difference in head position, ground pawing, use of the operated leg.
27	Dogs N=20-22	Ovariohysterectomy	Sham controls	Surgery group had increased sleep time, increased time in lateral recumbency, less time grooming, more time licking incision. Surgery group had fewer greeting behaviours (vocalising, door pawing, tail wagging, orienting, lip licking, attempting to escape) when the cage door was opened. On abdominal palpation, tag wagging and lip licking more frequent in controls. Arched back, vocalisation, abrupt head lifting and snarling were seen only during palpation of the abdomen of surgery dogs; no significant difference from controls.

Table 4
Examples of acute pain behaviours documented by comparison between animals treated with an analgesic and animals treated with placebo after surgery

Reference number	Species group size	Procedure	Analgesic	Effect of analgesic
25	Rats N=8-10	Nephrectomy, jugular cutdown	Nalbuphine, various doses	Highest dose prevented decrease in locomotor activity, partially prevented decrease in food and water consumption
28	Rats N=8-9	Flank laparotomy	Buprenorphine, various doses	Body weight loss significantly different from controls in all dose groups, all doses prevented decrease in water consumption, one dose prevented decrease in food consumption
29	Dogs N=13-14	Ovariohysterectomy	Carprofen, one dose, given pre- or post-operatively	Lower pain scores in pre-operative group for 8 h after surgery. Pain score was a visual analogue assessment scoring overall response to interaction, handling and palpation of the surgical wound.
30	Cats N=42 (21 controls)	Onychectomy	Butorphanol	Pain, appetite, personality and lameness scores lower in treated animals for 2 days after surgery. Five point descriptive scales were collapsed to 2 point scales to show significant differences.
31	Cats N=10	Ovariohysterectomy	Medetomidine / ketamine*	Pain scores lower for 18 hours after surgery. Five point descriptive scales were collapsed to 2 point scales to show significant differences.

* Controls received acepromazine/thiopentone/halothane.

Pain scales

Despite the difficulties associated with grading pain behaviour, there have been numerous studies performed using pain scores or scales. There are four methods commonly used. The simple descriptive scale usually has 3-5 gradations and descriptions of what each number looks like (Figure 1).

A) 4 = non-weight bearing lameness,
     3 = marked lameness,
     2 = mild lameness,
     1 = intermittent lameness,
     0 = normal gait

B) 4 = Worst possible pain. Looks uncomfortable and cannot touch wound. Growl and hiss.
     3 = Looks uncomfortable but can touch wound.
     2 = Happy cat, flinch on wound stroke.
     1 = Happy cat, purr and friendly. Flinch with wound pressure, but not with stroke over area.
     0 = No pain.

C) 3 = severe pain,
     2 = moderate pain,
     1 = mild pain,
     0 – no pain.

Figure 1 Examples of simple descriptive scales [31,34,35].

The observer watches the animal and picks a number. Visual analogue scales are standard length lines that have no pain at one end and worst pain ever at the other (Fig. 2).

No pain_____Worst pain imaginable

Sound_____Could not be more lame

Figure 2 Examples of visual analogue scales [34,36].

There are often behavioural descriptions of what the two ends of the line look like. The observer draws a line at the point they judge the pain to be. The distance from no pain to the mark is divided by the total length of the line, giving a pain score. A numerical rating scale is similar, except that the observer picks a number from 0-10 or 0-100 (Fig. 3).

No pain	0	1	2	3	4	5	6	7	8	9	10	Worst pain imaginable

Figure 3 Example of a numerical rating [35].

The above scales all require that the observer watch the animal and decide on a single number that provides a global judgment of the pain the animal is experiencing. Another approach is to construct a pain score from many variables [37,38]. Physiological variables are often incorporated into these scores, although they can be based on behaviour alone. Sometimes, individual variables are given different weights in the calculation of the final score. The observer does not know what the total score will be, but simply records values for each variable (Fig. 4).

Confusingly, this method of scoring has also been called a numerical rating scale. For purposes of clarity in this discussion, these scales will be called variable rating scales.

Recently, attempts have been made to compare various methods of generating a pain score and assessing pain. Conzemius et al. compared a visual analogue scale and a three variable rating scale to heart rate, respiratory rate, blood pressure and a mechanical pain threshold test as methods for judging pain after surgery to repair ruptured cranial cruciate ligaments in dogs [39]. The three variables in the rating scale were vocalisation, movement and agitation. Both the visual analogue scale and the variable rating scale correlated poorly with objective variables, but did correlate with each other and the amount of vocalisation. Holton and coworkers compared a simple descriptive scale, a numerical rating scale and a visual analogue scale for rating

University of Melbourne Pain Scale		
Category	Descriptor	Score
Physiologic data		0
a)	Physiologic data within reference range	
b)	Dilated pupils	2
c) *Choose only one*	Percentage increase in heart rate relative to preprocedural rate	
	>20%	1
	>50%	2
	>100%	3
d) *Choose only one*	Percentage increase in respiratory rate relative to preprocedural rate	
	>20%	1
	>50%	2
	>100%	3
e)	Rectal temperature exceeds reference range	1
f)	Salivation	2
Response to palpation		
Choose only one	No change from preprocedural behaviour	0
	Guards/reacts* when touched	2
	Guards/reacts* before touched	3
Activity		
Choose only one	At rest -steeping	0
	-semiconscious	0
	-awake	1
	Eating	0
	Restless (pacing continuously, getting up and down)	2
	Rolling, thrasing	3
Mental status		
Choose only one	Submissive	0
	Overtly friendly	1
	Wary	2
	Aggressive	3
Posture		
a)	Guarding or protecting affected area (includes fetal position)	2
b) *Choose only one*	Lateral recumbency	0
	Sternal recumbency	1
	Sitting or standing, head up	1
	Standing, head hanging down	2
	Moving	1
	Abnormal posture (eg, prayer position, hunched back)	2
Vocalisation **		
Choose only one	Not vocalising	0
	Vocalising when touched	2
	Intermittent vocalisation	2
	Continuous vocalisation	3

The pain scale includes 6 categories. Each category contains descriptors of various behaviours that are assigned numeric values. The assessor examines the descriptors in each category and decides whether a descriptor approximates the dog's behaviour. If so, the value for that descriptor is added to the patient's pain score. Certain descriptors are mutually exclusive (eg, a dog cannot be in sternal recumbency and standing up at the same time).These mutually exclusive descriptors are grouped together with the notation "choose only one". For category 4, mental status, the assessor must have completed a preprocedural assessment of the dog's dominant/aggressive behavior to establish a baseline score. The mental status score is the absolute difference between preprocedural and postprocedural scores. The minimum possible total pain score is 0 points, the maximum total pain score is 27 points.

*   Includes turning head toward affected area; or tense muscles and a protective (guarding) posture.
**   Does not include alert barking.

Reprinted with permission, JAVMA 1999;214:658.

Figure 4 *Example of a variable rating scale [38].*

pain after various surgeries in dogs [35]. Four observers scored 50 dogs. The variability between observers and the variability between the observers and the dogs accounted for 29-36% of the total variability. There was only fair agreement among observers. The authors suggested that a 0-10 numerical rating scale, used by a single observer, might represent the best method for reducing variability, yet retain some method of grading animal pain.

In a fairly rigorous attempt to validate a variable rating scale for dogs, Firth and Haldane compared 36 dogs undergoing anaesthesia and ovariohysterectomy to 12 dogs undergoing anaesthesia alone [38]. The variable rating scale had 6 categories (physiological data, response to palpation, activity, mental status, posture, and vocalisation) and a total of 12 variables. The anaesthetic regime provided minimal analgesia and the dogs were divided into groups of 6 dogs that were give no analgesic drugs, butorphanol or carprofen. A blinded observer scored the dogs. The dogs were also videotaped at the time of scoring. The videotapes were scrambled and scored by a second observer. The scale showed clear discrimination between dogs that were anaesthetised and dogs that were anaesthetized and had surgery. All categories except activity demonstrated differences between the dogs that had surgery and those that did not have surgery. The scale also allowed discrimination within the various surgery treatment groups and the differences followed the expected time courses for the drugs used. The categories that showed the most differences within the dogs undergoing surgery were mental status and posture. Over the entire population, there was excellent agreement between observers on the score. For an individual dog, however, the observers could differ by as much as 4.5 points in either direction, while the difference between dogs that were anaesthetized and dogs that were anaesthetized and had surgery was 3.4 points.

Chronic pain

Detailed observations of the behaviours associated with chronic pain in animals are rare. Most studies involve assessment of lameness and assume that the lameness is secondary to pain in the lame limb.

Welsh, Gettinby and Nolan compared a visual analogue scale (sound——could not be more lame) to a simple descriptive scale (0=clinically sound, 1=barely detectable lameness, 2=obvious lameness, 3=severe head nod and possibly resting foot when standing, 4=carrying leg at trot) in the assessment of sheep with footrot [36]. Both scales showed good agreement between 2 observers, but were not interchangeable. Variability was highest when judging moderately lame sheep.

In comparisons between objective measurements of lameness using force plate analysis and subjective measurements using either simple descriptive scales or a variable rating scale, human observers were able to judge large differences in lameness in dogs, and were better at detecting differences in the stifle than in the hip [34,40]. In a study evaluating the efficacy of the analgesic etodolac in dogs with hip dysplasia, observers could not differentiate lack of improvement from improvements of 4-12% measured by forceplate [40]. Interestingly, all dogs were judged to improve with treatment, suggesting that the placebo effect was high. In a study evaluating long term recovery after total hip replacement, lameness scores improved by one month after surgery, while ground reaction forces did not improve until three months after surgery [34]. Once again, a placebo effect appeared to be present. Overall, subjective scores predicted only 60% of the objective data.

In a study evaluating the ability of human observers to detect signs of chronic pain in mice with gallstones, no differences from unaffected mice were noted in behaviour within a group, exploratory behaviour, stance, hair coat, position of the eyes, discharge from eyes and nose, cleanliness of the anal orifice, or condition of the tail [41]. The affected mice did squeak more readily than unaffected mice when the cranial abdomen was palpated. Injection of sodium urate into joints has been used to study the behaviour of painful chickens. (Gouty arthritis is commonly seen in caged meat birds and chronic pain can be a welfare issue). Sitting, standing on one leg, and limping are all increased in the birds with arthritis, while standing on two legs, walking, pecking at food, pecking the environment, pacing, scratching, preening, vocalisation and drinking do not differ between birds with and without arthritis [42].

Observer biases

How discriminating can humans be when attempting to assess animal pain using behavioural clues? Studies have shown that although adult humans can use 100 point scales, most actually self-report 11-21 levels of pain [43]. Children can self-report 6 levels of pain using a picture scale [44]. The question of how many levels of pain can be distinguished when adult humans observe other adult humans, children or animals has not been well studied. The branding studies in cattle and the castration/tail docking studies in lambs showed that, with quantitative counts of behaviour, 3-4 levels of pain could be described [19-22]. Similarly, 3-4 different doses of morphine could be distinguished in the hot plate test or formalin test, particularly if multiple behaviours were combined to create a composite score [6,10,13]. The force plate data indicated that observers could not distinguish differences in hip lameness when the changes in weight-bearing were less than 15%, which would suggest that, at most, 6 grades of lameness can be detected [40]. Studies of human emergency room physicians have shown it takes a 18 mm change on a 100 mm visual analogue scale before the doctor will indicate that there is a 'little more' or 'little less' pain [45]. It may be no accident that most simple descriptive scales use 3-5 grades of pain or lameness.

In addition to being realistic about how finely the human observer can grade animal pain behaviour, it behoves the caretaker to be aware of observational biases. Humans have an innate sensitivity to sounds similar to a human infant's cry and, without training, will provide care and grade pain based largely on vocalisations and extreme behavioural manifestations of pain [46-48]. Even when we use appropriate behaviours to measure animal pain, the placebo effect may occur if we anticipate that a treatment ought to provide relief [34,40]. This may be particularly true if the differences in pain behaviour are at the edge of our observational ability or are badly confounded by large genetic differences within the population under observation.

Conclusion

The question of what animal pain behaviour looks like and how human observers respond to and scale that behaviour is not trivial. The development of rational animal welfare laws, humane husbandry practices, and effective analgesic regimes for animals depends on accurate behavioural descriptions. The study of pain physiology uses behaviour as the measure of pain, even when the gene for the number of opiate receptors being expressed on a neuron is the subject of study.

Within genetically variable clinic populations, it is probably wise to score animals as 'comfortable' or 'uncomfortable', particularly if multiple, unblinded observers are used. Trained, blinded observers, using validated variable rating scales, can probably distinguish between two treatment groups in addition to a placebo group, assuming major differences between treatments. The use of a single blinded observer, videotapes, quantitative behavioural measures or a validated variable rating scale incorporating multiple behaviours should allow 5-6 levels of pain to be measured with reasonable group sizes (5-10 genetically similar same sex animals, 15-20 genetically dissimilar same sex animals).

The difficulty of measuring behaviour has lead many clinical researchers to abandon behavioural pain measurement and to use quantitative outcome variables, rather than behaviour, to assess pain. Examples are force plate measurements of weightbearing, time to walking, total locomotor activity, total food consumption, time to resumption of feeding, weight loss or gain, and number of days in the hospital for a given surgical procedure. There is no doubt that these variables measure an outcome of a given treatment and the outcome most certainly relates to pain in many instances. However, unless the outcome measurement tool is easily adapted to use in an individual patient by busy clinicians, these measurements will not help in the clinical assessment of pain.

Where does this leave the individual caretaker trying to use behaviour to assess the pain level of an individual patient at an individual time point? With training, we can tone down our reliance on vocalisations and extreme behaviour and increase our sensitivity to silent evidence of suffering. However, the placebo effect is almost impossible to avoid in this situation: we want that animal not to suffer. This suggests that global assessment is likely to be biased. Use of a variable rating scale, validated for species specific behaviours, that forces treatment when a certain score is reached, may be the most accurate method of assuring treatment in a clinical setting.

References

1   Mogil JS, Sternberg WF, Marek P, Sadowski B, Belknap JK, Leibeskind JC. The genetics of pain and pain inhibition. Proc Natl Acad Sci. USA 1996;93:3048-55.

2   Aliosi AM, Sacerdote P, Albonetti ME, Carli G. Sex-related effects on behaviour and B-endorphin of different intensities of formalin pain in rats. Brain Research 1995;699:242-9.

3   Cook CJ, Maasland SA, Devine CE. Social behaviour in sheep relates to behaviour and neurotransmitter responses to nociceptive stimuli. Physiology Behaviour 1996;60:741-51.

4   Sanford J, Ewbank R, Molony V, Tavernor WD, Urarov O. Guidelines for recognition and assessment of pain in animals. Vet Rec 1986;118:334-8.

5   Ramzan I, Wong BK, Corcoran GB. Pain sensitivity in dietary-induced obese rats. Physiology Behaviour 1993;54:433-5.

6   Espejo EF, Stinus L, Cador M, Mir D. Effects of morphine and naloxone on behaviour in the hot plate test: an ethopharmacological study in the rat. Psychopharmacology 1994;113:500-10.

7   Bowd AD. Ethics and animals experimentation. American Psychologist 1980;35:224-5.

8   Dubner R. Methods of assessing pain in animals. In: Wall PD, Melzack R. Textbook of Pain, 3rd edn. Edinburgh: Churchill Livingstone, 1994:293-302.

9   Espejo EF, Mir D. Structure of the rat's behaviour in the hot plate test. Behav Brain Res 1993;56:171-6.

10 Belknap JK, Lame M, Danielson PW. Inbred strain differences in morphine-induced analgesia with the hot plate assay: a reassessment. Behav Genetics 1990;20:333-8.

11 Ness TJ, Gebhart GF. Colorectal distention as a noxious visceral stimulus: physiologic and pharmacologic characterization of pseudoaffective reflexes in the rat. Brain Res 1988;450:153-69.

12 Pippi NL, Lumb WV, Fialho SAG, Scott RJ. J Equine Med Surg 1979;3:430-5.

13 Abbott FV, Franklin KBJ, Westbrook RF. The formalin test: scoring properties of the first and second phases of the pain response in rats. Pain 1995;60:91-102.

14 Sora I, Li X, Funada M, Kinsey S, Uhl GR. Visceral chemical nociception in mice lacking mu-opioid receptors: effects of morphine, SNC80 and U-50,488. Eur J Pharmacol 1999;366:R3-R5.

15 Attal N, Filliatreau G, Perrot S, Jazat F, Di Giamberardino L, Guilbaud G. Behavioural pain-related disorders and contribution of the saphenous nerve in crush and chronic constriction injury of the rat sciatic nerve. Pain 1994;59:301-12.

16 Morton DB, Griffiths PHM. Guidelines on the recognition of pain, distress and discomfort in experimental animals and an hypothesis for treatment. Vet Rec 1985;116:431-6.

17 American College of Veterinary Anesthesiologists. American College of Veterinary Anesthesiologists' position paper on the treatment of pain in animals. JAVMA 1998;213:628-30.

18 Flecknell PA. Assessment of pain. In: Flecknell PA. Laboratory Animal Anesthesia, 2nd edn. Academic Press–Harcourt Brace, London, 1996:138-43.

19 Lay Jr DC, Friend TH, Bowers CL, Grissom KK, Jenkins OC. A Comparative physiological and behavioural study of freeze and hot-iron branding using dairy cows. J Anim Sci 1992;70:1121-25.

20 Lay Jr DC, Friend TH, Grissom KK, Bowers CL, Mal ME. Effects of freeze or hot-iron branding of Angus calves on some physiological and behavioural indicators of stress. App Anim Behav 1992;33:137-47.

21 Schwartzkopf-Genswein KS, Stookey JM, Welford R. Behaviour of cattle during hot-iron and freeze branding and the effects on subsequent handling ease. J Anim Sci 1997;75:2064-72.

22 Kent JE, Molony V, Robertson IS. Comparison of the Burdizzo and rubber ring methods for castrating and tail docking lambs. Vet Rec 1995;136:192-6.

23 Jansen van 't Land C, Hendriksen CFM. Change in locomotor activity pattern in mice: a model for recognition of distress. Lab Animals 1995;29:286-93.

24 Farr La, Campbell-Grossman C, Mack JM. Circadian disruption and surgical recovery. Nurs Res 1988;37:170-5.

25 Flecknell PA, Liles JH. The effects of surgical procedures, halothane anaesthesia and nalbuphine on locomotor activity and food and water consumption in rats. Lab Animals 1991;25:50-60.

26 Raekallio M, Taylor PM, Bloomfield M. A comparison of methods for evaluation of pain and distress after orthopaedic surgery in horses. J Vet Anaesth 1997;24:17-20.

27 Hardie EM, Hansen BD. Behaviour after ovariohysterectomy in the dog: what's normal? App Anim Behav Sci 1997;51:111-28.

28 Flecknell PA, Roughan JV, Stewart R. Use of oral buprenorphine ('buprenorphine jello')for postoperative analgesia in rats-aclinical trial. Lab Animals 1999;33:169-74.

29 Lascelles Bd, Cripps PJ, Jones A, Waterman-Pearson A. Efficacy and kinetics of carprofen, administered preoperatively or postoperatively, for the prevention of pain in dogs undergoing ovariohysterectomy. Vet Surg 1998;27:568-82.

30 Carroll GL, Howe LB, Slater MR, Haughn L, Martinez EA, Hartsfield SM, Mathews NS. Evaluation of analgesia provided by postoperative butorphanol to cats undergoing onychectomy. J Am Vet Med Assoc 1998;213:246-50.

31 Slingsby LS, Lane EC, Mears ER, Shanson MC, Waterman-Pearson AE. Postoperative pain after ovariohysterectomy in the cat: a comparison of two anesthetic regimens. Vet Rec 1998;143:589-90.

32 Slingsby LS, Waterman-Pearson AE. Comparison of pethidine, buprenorphine and ketoprofen for postoperative analgesia after ovariohysterectomy in the cat. Vet Rec 1998;143:185-9.

33 Flecknell PA, Orr HE, Roughan JV, Stewart R. Comparison of the effects of oral or subcutaneous carprofen or ketoprofen in rats undergoing laparotomy. Vet Rec 1999;144:65-7.

34 Budsberg SC, Chambers JN, Van Lue SL, Foutz TL, Reece L. Prospective evaluation of ground reaction forces in dogs undergoing unilateral total hip replacement. Am J Vet Res 1996;57:1781-5.

35 Holton LL, Scott EM, Nolan AM, Reid J, Welsh E, Flaherty D. Comparison of three methods used for assessment of pain in dogs. J Am Vet Med Assoc 1998;212:61-6.

36 Welsh EM, Gettinby G, Nolan AM. Comparison of a visual analog scale and a numerical rating scale for assessment of lameness, using sheep as the model. Am J Vet Res 1993;54:976-84.

37 Winkler KP, Greenfield CL, Benson GJ. The effect of wound irrigation with bupivicaine on postoperative analgesia of the feline onychectomy patient. J Am Anim Hosp Assoc. 1997;33:346-52.

38 Firth AM, Haldane SL. Development of a scale to evaluate postoperative pain in dogs. J Am Vet Med Assoc 1999;214:651-9.

39 Conzemius MG, Hill CM, Sammarco JL, Perowski SZ. Correlation between subjective and objective measures used to determine severity of postoperative pain in dogs. J Am Vet Med Assoc 1997;210:210-22.

40 Budsberg Sc, Johnston SA, Schwarz PD, DeCamp CE, Claxton R. Efficacy of etodolac for the treatment of osteoarthritis of the hip joints in dogs. J Am Vet Med Assoc 1999;214:206-10.

41 Beynen AC, Baumann V, Bertens APMG, Hesp APM, Van Zutphen FM. Assessment of discomfort in gallstone-bearing mice: a practical example of the problems encountered in an attempt to recognize discomfort in laboratory animals. Lab Animals 1987;21:35-42.

42 Wylie LM, Gentle MJ. Feeding-induced tonic pain suppression in the chicken: reversal by naloxone. Physiology Behaviour 1998;64:27-30.

43 Jensen MP, Turner JA, Romano JM. What is the maximum number of levels needed in pain intensity measurement? Pain 1994 Sep;58:387-92.

44 Chambers CT, McGrath PJ. Pain Measurement in Children. In Ashburn MA, Rice LJ (Eds). The Management of Pain. Churchill Livingstone, New York,1998:625-34.

45 Todd KH, Funk JP. The minimum clinically important difference in physician-assigned visual analog pain scores. Acad Emerg Med 1996 Feb;3:142-6.

46 Hansen B. Through a glass darkly: using behaviour to assess pain. Sem Vet Med 1997;12:61-74.

47 Zeskind PS, Sale J, Maio L, Huntington L, Weiseman JR. Adult perception of pain and hunger cries: a synchrony of arousal. Child Development 1985;56:549-54.

48 Chambers CT, Reid GJ, Craig KD, McGrath PJ, Finley GA. Agreement between child and parent reports of pain. Clin J Pain 1998;14:336-42.

5

PATHOPHYSIOLOGY OF PAIN IN ANIMALS AND ITS CONSEQUENCE FOR ANALGESIC THERAPY

Ludo J. Hellebrekers, DVM, PhD, DipECVA,
Faculty of Veterinary Medicine, Utrecht University, Utrecht,
The Netherlands

Introduction

In the attempt to unravel the pathophysiological background of pain one needs to introduce the term nociception, and differentiate this from the term pain. The *International Association for the Study of Pain* defined pain as being 'an unpleasant sensory or emotional experience associated with actual or potential tissue damage or described in terms of such damage'. Since *pain* relates to the way the unpleasant or aversive sensation is experienced by the individual, it would be more correct to limit the use of this term in animals.

The term *nociception* relates to the recognition of signals in the nervous system that originate in sensory receptors (*nociceptors*) and that provide information related to tissue damage. Despite this significant and relevant difference in definition, the term pain is used equally with regard to animals as well as humans, both within the veterinary community and by the lay public.

When nociceptors are stimulated, the free sensory nerve endings are activated and, depending on the type of stimulation, the action potential will be transported centrally by a specific class of fibres. Nociceptors that respond to thermal or mechanical stimulation have small diameter; they are myelinated fibres (Aδ-type) that transport at high speed (5-30 m/s) and in humans are known to be related to a sharp pain sensation and are involved in the reflex withdrawal response.

The other group of nociceptors are labelled polymodal nociceptors, which can be stimulated, in a variety of ways, such as by stimuli of a chemical or intense thermal (hot or cold) or mechanical nature. The signals from these receptors are transported by afferent fibres of a different class (C-type fibres), being of a small diameter, and unmyelinated, with a conduction velocity of 0.5-2 m/s.

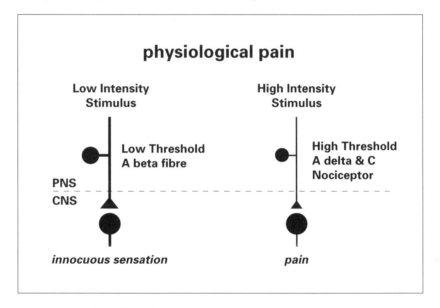

Figure 1 Physiological pain
In 'physiological' conditions the low-intensity stimulation results in a non-noxious (tactile) stimulus, while the high-intensity stimulus, following activation of the nociceptor and propagation of the signal by separate afferent pathways, may lead to pain.
PNS – peripheral nervous system;
CNS – central nervous system
From: Woolf and Chong, Anesth Analg 1993;77:372-379

Upon activation, these C-type fibres will intensify the original stimulus activity and be responsible for the dull, longer-lasting pain.

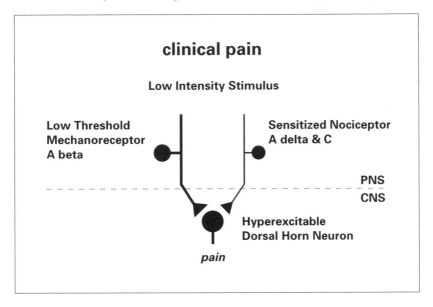

Figure 2 Clinical pain
In a pain state, the change in PNS and CNS processing of the sensory information, and subsequent hyperexcitability, results in low-intensity stimuli now being perceived as painful.
PNS – peripheral nervous system; CNS – central nervous system
From: Woolf and Chong, Anesth Analg 1993;77:372-379

Whereas this, rather simplified, presentation may hold true under situations of short duration stimulation, other types of neural structures have been recognised over the years as being able to relay painful stimuli. These include, among others, so-called 'sleeping nociceptors' that may become active and able to transport signals following a (relatively short, of the order of hours) period of inflammation. The change of these 'sleeping nociceptors' to an active state may even result in clear response to an innocuous stimulation, thereby providing the first element of peripheral sensitisation (see later).

It is this knowledge that makes it obvious that within pain physiology there is no stable, pre-determined stimulus-response relationship. The final and total response to nociceptor stimulation depends not only on the intensity and duration of stimulation but also on the pre-existing state of activity of those elements of the neural system involved in the perception and processing of this stimulation.

From the periphery, the afferent fibres enter the spinal canal as peripheral nerves through the dorsal root, into the dorsal horn of the spinal cord where the further processing of the signals takes place.

The Aδ-fibres, for instance, connect through interneurons with motor neurons that are responsible for the reflex withdrawal response. Next to these (inter)segmental reflexes, sensory information relevant to pain sensation is relayed through specific pathways to distinct areas of the brain such as the thalamic region and the reticular formation. From here onward the information is relayed to the sensory cortex where the conscious experience takes place.

Next to the transport of sensory information from the periphery to higher structures in the central nervous system, extensive processing of the sensory information takes place at different levels of the central nervous system. Locally, at the level of the spinal cord, as well as through descending tracts originating from the medulla, modulation and processing of sensory information will take a form depending on circumstances and overall level of activity.

Peripheral sensitisation

Following the initial stimulation of the nociceptor the propagation of the activity will take place along specific fibres, the type of which depends on the character and origin of the stimulus and the nociceptor type activated.

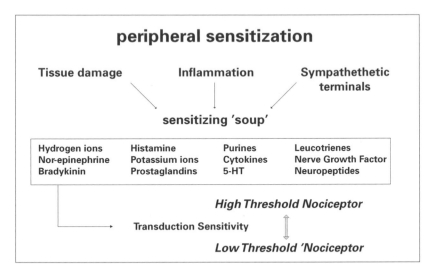

Figure 3 Peripheral sensitisation
Different primary events may create a sensitising environment around the peripheral nerve ending inducing an increased sensitivity thereof.
5-HT – 5 hydroxytryptamine
From: Woolf and Chong, Anesth Analg 1993;77:372-379

Mechanical and thermal nociceptor stimulation results in transport through Aδ-type afferent fibres whereas C-type fibres propagate activity originating from polymodal receptors.

Next to the primary process initiated with nociceptor activation, the same activation leads to a number of processes that determine the character and intensity of further responses to subsequent stimulation.

Following initial stimulation in the intact, not previously stimulated individual, it is the activation of the high threshold receptors by thermal or mechanical stimuli that leads to pain. When, due to the character of the initial injury or tissue damage, the stimulation is prolonged, the response pattern changes. The inflammatory processes accompanying the tissue trauma can primarily account for this change in response pattern, and subsequent sensitisation.

This phenomenon, called peripheral sensitisation, is largely dependent on the release of vasoactive amines from damaged tissue and inflammatory cells, and on the release of neuropeptides released from excited nociceptive nerve endings in the injured area.

These latter peptides further stimulate inflammatory cells to set free a whole spectrum of chemical inflammatory mediators, as a result of which the free nerve endings of the nociceptive afferents are 'bathed' in an environment of different kinds of inflammatory mediators. This 'inflammatory soup', consists of several vasoactive amines, ions, neuropeptides and different products of the arachidonic acid cycle. The exposition of the nociceptor to this inflammatory/-sensitising environment results in an increased sensitivity of the (originally) high-threshold nociceptors, to now respond to low-intensity stimuli. The consequence of this is that stimulation that was previously perceived as non-painful/innocuous now results in a painful experience.

Central sensitisation

Primary afferents from peripheral nociceptors enter the spinal cord and terminate in specific regions of the dorsal horn, connecting to fibres ascending to higher centres. Basically, afferent fibres terminate on either one of two classes of dorsal horn neurons, of which the 'high-threshold nociceptor-specific' neurons respond specifically to noxious stimuli. Under normal circumstances, the so-called 'wide dynamic range' neurons are responsive to non-noxious stimulation, processing this to be perceived as a tactile experience.

When stimulation persists in time, the wide dynamic range neurons become sensitised, leading to hyperresponsiveness. As a consequence, non-noxious stimulation will now result in a painful experience that in duration outlasts the original nociceptive input.

The activated wide dynamic range neurons can be held accountable for the increased sensitivity to mechanical stimulation as well as for the spread of the (hyper)sensitivity of the uninjured tissue surrounding the damaged region.

The changes in spinal processing (i.e. the central or spinal neuroplasticity) of sensory input results in a situation whereby pain is perceived upon stimuli entering the dorsal horn by way of low-threshold Aδ-afferent fibres that are normally not involved in the perception of pain. Furthermore, the increase in spinal excitability will be followed by spatial (receptive field), temporal (duration of stimulus and response) and threshold (sensitivity) increase, together resulting in a hypersensitive and hyperactive state at spinal level.

Also following deafferentation or denervation, spinal or central neuroplasticity is held responsible for the increased neuronal activity and is influenced by the level of noxious stimulation prior to the deafferentation. The unabated biting of animals on the insensate area, even to the point of automutilation, underscore the severity of the situation and support a rigorous approach of (local) analgesic therapy.

It has become clear from human as well as animal studies that for optimal results in reducing this stimulus-induced increase in

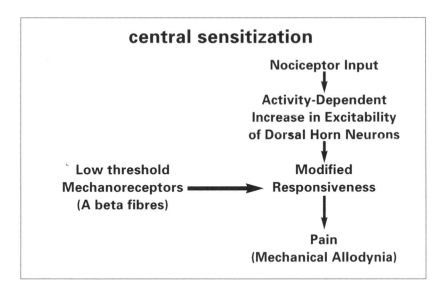

Figure 4 Central sensitisation
Prolonged exposure to noxious stimulation induces an increased level of sensitivity of the central nervous system and subsequently, low-intensity stimuli may become painful rather then innocuous (or non-painful). From: Woolf and Chong, Anesth Analg 1993;77:372-379

excitability at the spinal level, analgesics must be administered before rather then (shortly) after the start of stimulus. By an effective prevention of the development of hyperexcitability, a reduction of post-operative pain can be achieved long after the pharmacological duration of action of the analgesic drug.

Pathophysiology of pain and analgesic therapy - Peri-operative pain control

When do we need to treat pain?

The present insight into the pathophysiologic background of how and where the sensory signal originates and where it is processed, allow us multiple options to intervene in these processes in an attempt to achieve adequate pain relief. The question remains as to whether the presence of pain does not hold certain beneficial qualities that would be lost upon instalment of effective pain control. It is undeniably true that by exhibiting pain symptoms, it becomes easier to recognise and diagnose certain pathologies, especially those of the extremities. Furthermore, it can be stated that refraining from weight bearing in the case of a fractured leg, can indeed reduce the risk of further trauma.

Despite the above, it should be realised that a large number of negative aspects can be ascribed to the prolonged presence of pain, both in a physical as well as psychological sense. Therefore, overall treatment should always aim to achieve a situation whereby a compromise is reached between both negative and positive aspects.

An important aspect of this discussion lies in the fact that, except under conditions of general anaesthesia, full analgesia cannot be achieved by systemic administration of analgesic drugs such as opioids, alpha2-adrenergic agonists or Non-Steroidal Anti-Inflammatory Drugs (NSAIDs). As a consequence, a number of positive aspects remain intact (for instance the animal will still refrain from using the fractured leg) while at the same time the negative consequences of pain are kept to a minimum.

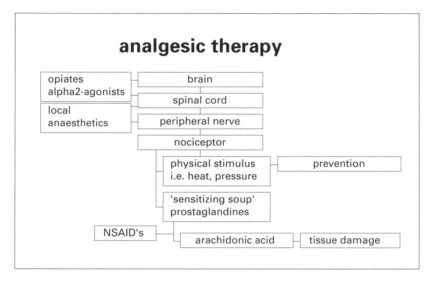

Figure 5 *Schematic presentation of pain pathway and potential therapeutic options for achieving pain relief.*

The negative consequences of pain are multiple in nature but can be grouped under the heading of 'stress-response'. As a consequence of this stress response, and next to the discomfort and impaired welfare of the animal, a number of physiological functions will be impaired. The animals are likely to get into a negative energy balance and research has shown that there is clear suppression of the immune status. As a result, wound healing will be slowed down, and the incidence of post-surgical complication increases. In the most serious of cases even automutilation is seen.

Research performed within the laboratory animal world has shown that when analgesics are excluded from the post-anaesthetic treatment protocol, the weight loss in the period immediately following surgery was greater than when adequate analgesic therapy was included. Due to the large variation in both the type of patients and interventions, these kinds of consequences are much more difficult to manage in clinical veterinary practice, despite the fact that there is every reason to assume that this applies to the patient population as well.

In conclusion, it can be stated that adequate pain relief promotes the animal's overall well-being as well as having a positive effect on the speed and quality of post-surgical recovery. At the same time, the positive aspects will be retained since pain treatment aims for, and achieves, a state whereby the pain will not be completely relieved but has become more endurable.

Prevention of pain is more effective than 'cure'

When taking into account the pathophysiological aspects discussed above, it becomes obvious that in order to prevent peripheral and central sensitisation from developing, one needs to provide sufficient analgesic therapy at a very early stage, to prevent the initial pain stimulus form occurring. Under clinical circumstances, this approach will not always be feasible, as for instance in trauma cases. In such cases, the lack of possibility of preventing the initial pain for a large part can be held accountable for relative ineffectiveness of subsequent pain therapy.

Prevention of pain not only relates to timely administration of analgesic drugs (for instance, the premedication before surgical anaesthesia) but also has clear implications for the design of the pain treatment protocol following (surgical) trauma. When, due to an inadequate dosage or too lengthy dosing intervals, the pain treatment is less then optimally effective, the sensory system will be activated with the probability that the final overall pain relief will be insufficient.

In pain treatment protocols, an important rule is that it is essential that treatment is installed on time, at an adequate dose and with correct dosing intervals in order in order to achieve an effective pain relief (see Fig. 6 A-D).

Therapeutic options

Especially when the demand for pain control concerns analgesia for elective surgical procedures, the importance of adequate (analgesic) premedication cannot be overestimated. It is obvious that adequate analgesia should be maintained during the surgical intervention as well, but the analgesic drug administered before the induction of anaesthesia can serve (depending on duration and severity of the procedure) as a basis for further maintenance of analgesia. To achieve analgesia under these conditions, one can choose between different classes of drugs, such as opioids or alpha2-adrenergic agonists. Traditionally, the analgesic component in the premedication of the dog has been an opioid drug, whereas in other species such as horses, cattle, and cats the alpha2-adrenergic agonists have been the primary analgesics.

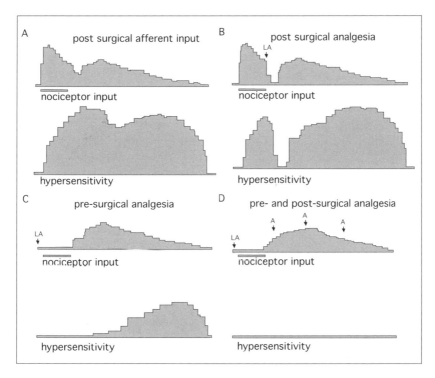

Figure 6A-D *The models in figures A–D depict the effect of prolonged nociceptor stimulation without analgesic therapy (A) on the development of hypersensitivity; the short-duration effect of the single administration of a local anaesthetic (LA) either post-operatively (B) or pre-operatively (C) and ultimately the proposed effect on the development of hypersensitivity of adequate pre-operative analgesic blockade followed by repeated analgesic administration post-operatively (D).*
From: Woolf and Chong, Anesth Analg 1993;77:372-379

With the development of newer drugs within the aforementioned classes, as well as with gaining more insight into possibilities for existing drugs in different species, the options have become more variable. Both classes of drugs provide a good basis for obtaining surgical analgesia and, together with other anaesthetic drugs, achieving general anaesthesia. Although the duration of action in many instances will be adequately long, repeat administration may be indicated when short-acting drugs such as fentanyl are used, or when the procedure extends to more then 60 minutes.

Next to the aforementioned opioids and alpha2-adrenergic agonists, another approach to pain relief in the peri-operative period includes the application of NSAIDs. This class of drugs has traditionally been used in the treatment of chronic, and specifically orthopaedic, pain. The primary reason that limited the use of these drugs pre- and per-operatively was related to their mechanism of action. The class of NSAIDs inhibit the formation of prostaglandins that play a crucial role in the development of pain. This inhibition however also extends to those prostaglandins that play a regulatory role in the determination of renal perfusion and functioning of the intestinal tract. The combination of the application of these drugs under conditions of reduced perfusion (as can be seen as a consequence of anaesthesia) could easily induce serious complications, especially regarding renal function. Newer drugs, with a slightly different spectrum of activity and a greater safety margin could potentially overcome these objections to the pre- and per-operative use of NSAIDs and allow for a truly multimodal design of analgesic therapy.

Bibliography

1   Coderre TJ, Katz J, Vaccarino AL, Melzack R. Contribution of central neuroplasticity to pathological pain: review of clinical and experimental evidence. Pain 1993;52:259-85.
2   Jessell TM, Kelly DD. Pain and analgesia. In: Principles of Neuroscience, 3rd edn. Kandel ER, Schwartz JH, Jessell TM (Eds), Prentice Hall, London, UK 1991:Chap27.

3 Lascelles BDX, Crêpes PJ, Jones A, Waterman AE. Post-operative central hypersensitivity and pain: the pre-emptive value of pethidine for ovariohysterectomie. Pain 1997;73:461-71.

4 O'Connor TC, Abram SE. Inhibition of nociception-induced spinal sensitisation by anesthetic agents. Anesthesiology 1995;82:259-66.

5 Sidle PJ, Cousins MJ. Introduction to pain mechanisms: implications for neural blockade. In: Neural Blockade in Clinical Anaesthesia and Management of Pain, 3rd edn. Cousins MJ, Bridenbaugh PO (Eds).Lippincott-Raven, New York 1998:Chap23,1.

6 Woolf CJ, Chong MS. Pre-emptive analgesia - Treating post-operative pain by preventing the establishment of central sensitisation. Ernest Analg 1993;77:372-9.

7 Yashpal K, Katz J, Coderre TJ. Effects of pre-emptive or post-injury intrathecal local anesthesia on persistent nociceptive responses in rats. Anesthesiology 1996;84:1119-28.

6

CLINICAL PHARMACOLOGY OF ANALGESIC AGENTS

B Duncan X Lascelles, *BSc BVSc PhD MRCVS CertVA*
DSAS(Soft Tissue) DipECVS, Department of Clinical Veterinary Science,
University of Bristol, Langford, UK

Introduction

Animal studies directly relating to pain have been carried out for nearly two thousand years. Galen, after studying the work of the Alexandrian anatomists Herophilus (335-280 BC) and Erasistratus (310-250 BC), re-established the importance of the central and peripheral nervous systems and their relationship to sensation and pain. However, only in the last two decades have real advances been made in understanding pain mechanisms and implementing effective therapy. In the late 1960s, there was the proposal of the 'gate theory'. This event sparked an exponential increase in the number of scientists working on pain and recently there has been a move to include psychologists and behavioural scientists in pain research. In the 1970s there was the discovery of endogenous opioid receptors and from there an explosion in pharmacological research in analgesics. Since that time, a progressive understanding of the physiology and pharmacology of pain, and the pharmacology of analgesics has led to an increasingly effective use of analgesics in the clinics. This chapter reviews the clinical pharmacology of common analgesic agents used in companion animals.

Drugs that are used as analgesics:
- *opioids*
- *local anaesthetics*
- *NSAID's*
- *alpha$_2$ adrenoceptor agonists*
- *dissociative agents (ketamine)*
- *inhalational agents (nitrous oxide)*
- *benzodiazapenes*

Opioids

Opioid drugs have been used to provide analgesia for over 2000 years. Opiates are drugs derived from opium, such as morphine and codeine, and opioids are drugs that act at opioid receptors. In the 1970s, opioid binding sites were identified in mammalian brain, and opioid receptors identified as μ, δ and κ. In the 1980s, pharmacological studies suggested the presence of subtypes of the μ- and κ-receptor. Cloning studies have not so far provided support for opioid receptor subtypes, but have identified other related genes such as the 'orphan' receptor (65% sequence homology to the other receptors). Opioid receptors have recently been reclassified as OP3 (μ), OP1 (δ) and OP2 (κ). Currently, the possibility of subtypes does not seem to be clinically relevant, and further discussion will use the original nomenclature of μ, δ and κ.

These receptors can have both excitatory and depressive effects and the balance between stimulation (increased locomotion, vocalisation, manic behaviour) and depression (analgesia, respiratory depression, sedation) is variable and there is a great deal of species variation.
Endogenous ligands exist for these receptors - the peptides β-endorphin, leu-enkephalin, met-enkephalin and dynorphin. They have different selectivities for the various receptors and also, depending on the relative quantities and conditions under which they are released, can produce analgesia or hyperalgesia, as well as having a variety of other effects throughout the body.

Opioids block the transmission of noxious stimuli to higher centres by acting on pre- and post-synaptic receptors [μ(OP3), δ(OP1) or κ(OP2)] of the primary afferent sensory nerve at the level of the spinal cord. They also act at higher 'centres' to produce analgesia. Opioids also act peripherally at opioid receptors that are generated in inflammatory conditions.

The concept of opioid/receptor interaction is often difficult to grasp but three main processes are involved:
1   *selectivity of opioid drug for receptor types*

2 *intrinsic activity or effect at the receptor(s)*

3 *affinity for the receptor*

Opioid drugs may be active at one, two or all of the receptors, and differences in drug selectivity may be used to predict some of the pharmacological properties. For example, μ-selective agonists produce analgesia and euphoria in humans and positive reinforcement in animals, whereas κ-selective agonists produce analgesia and dysphoria in humans but are highly aversive in animals.

Table 1

Selectivity of opioid drugs used in companion animals

	μ	κ	δ
Morphine	+++	+/-	+/-
Pethidine	++	-	-
Fentanyl	+++	-	-
Etorphine	+++	++	++
Buprenorphine	+++	++	+/-
Butorphanol	++	++	-
Nalbuphine	+	++	+
Naloxone	+++	+	+

This table shows the selectivity of the drugs for the various receptors, however their actions at these receptors can be agonist, partial agonist or antagonist (see main text)

Table 1 summarises the selectivity of opioid drugs used in companion animals. In terms of their intrinsic activity, expressed simplistically, drugs may range in activity from being pure agonists to pure antagonists. There are also drugs which fall into the continuum between these two extremes which are classified as partial agonists or agonist/antagonists (see Table 2).

Clinically, the most important distinction is between the pure agonists and the partial agonists or agonist/antagonists which may have a ceiling effect. The 'ceiling effect' is where the maximal effect produced at a particular dose is not increased by increasing the dose;

Table 2
Simple classification of common opioid drugs used in small companion
animals.

Agonists	Morphine
	Pethidine
	Oxymorphone
	Methadone
	Fentanyl
Mixed agonist-antagonists	Pentazocine
	Butorphanol
	Nalbuphine
Partial agonists	Buprenorphine
Antagonists	Naloxone
	Naltrexone

instead, as the dose is increased, antagonism of the effects can result
(the so-called 'bell shaped' dose response curve). This aspect is
discussed more fully later.

Also important clinically is the affinity for the receptor, with drugs
such as buprenorphine having a long duration of action due to the
high affinity for the receptor.

Other pharmacology of relevance clinically is the lipophilicity of
the drug (high lipid solubility can contribute to a long duration of
action) and potency. Potency however, is of little clinical relevance in
companion animals where the volume of injectate never limits the
amount of drug that can be administered. It is much more relevant
when one is considering the chemical control of wild animals that
have to be darted.

General clinical pharmacological actions of opioid drugs

The opioid drugs are fascinating in that they appear to have one pharmacology for when they are used in the presence of pain, and another for when they are not. The spectrum and severity of side effects is also very different between man and animals. These two factors have resulted in a number of 'myths' that have built up surrounding their clinical use, and very often are the reasons, unjustly, for the drugs being withheld. When combined with analgesics of other classes, the combined effect is often supra-additive. Therefore it is now recommended that opioids be used as early as possible and in combination with either local anaesthetics or NSAIDS. This is discussed more fully later.

Analgesia

All opioids act to block the transmission of noxious stimuli to higher centres by acting on receptors located pre- or post-synaptically at the primary afferent sensory nerve at the level of the spinal cord. They also act at higher centres to block the transmission of stimuli and to increase the amount of descending inhibitory influences (e.g. catecholaminergic system). Analgesia is produced by the drug's agonist activity at μ-, δ- and κ-receptor subtypes, and the degree of analgesia depends on the affinity and the intrinsic activity. The most predictable analgesia is obtained by the use of μ-selective agonists such as morphine, pethidine and fentanyl. However, all of the mentioned opioid drugs are good analgesics, but due to their individual properties, one drug may be more appropriate than another in a given situation.

A very important point is that the opioids need to be titrated against pain. If opioids are given according to the often-quoted 'duration of actions' of the various drugs, pain will be left untreated. The quoted 'duration of action' for a given drug should be taken as an approximate guide, and the patient reassessed at regular intervals.

Opioids can also act peripherally, as opioid receptors are produced peripherally in inflammatory states - on nerve endings and on inflammatory cells. The peripheral analgesic effects are apparent quite quickly following administration, and the peripheral effect can be made use of by administering the drug peripherally and so decreasing the potential for systemic side effects.

Sedation

Opioids produce sedation and are often used for their sedative effects. Dogs show sedation and a decrease in spontaneous locomotor activity. Sedation is often viewed as undesirable post-operatively, and thus opioids are often withheld. By using opioid drugs pre-operatively at appropriate doses, the central nervous system can be 'protected' from the adverse changes that occur as a result of noxious stimuli input (see previous chapter): smaller doses will then be needed post-operatively and so less sedation will be seen. Sedation is particularly marked with butorphanol, pethidine and morphine.

Excitement and use in felidae

Much of the notorious reputation of opiates in cats resulted from its use in gross overdose based entirely on the work of Joel and Arndts (1925) [1] who used a morphine dose of 20 mg/kg. Although clinical doses of opiates do not cause sedation in cats as is seen in dogs, they do not cause excitement or mania. However, it is probably unwise to use opioids by the intravenous route in conscious cats as temporary overstimulation of the CNS can be seen.

Excitement and use in equidae

Hyperexcitability in response to opioids, especially morphine, can occur in horses. Excitement may be related to individual susceptibility, and in part depends on the administered dose, excitement being minimal and possibly absent at low dose levels. However, μ-agonist opioids administered to horses in pain invariably calm the animal down. Other opioids such as butorphanol can cause box walking and excitement-type behaviour even in moderate doses. Other behaviours reported are compulsive eating and agitation.

Respiratory depression

Opioids, particularly the μ-selective drugs, produce respiratory depression by causing a decrease in the sensitivity of neurones in the medulla to CO_2 (in the conscious animal), and a delayed response of the respiratory centre. This is seen as a decrease in respiratory rate with little change in tidal volume. Partial agonists produce less respiratory depression and there is a 'ceiling' to this effect. But respiratory depression is not a feature of use of opioids in animals unless very high doses are used and the animal is not in pain, or if opioids are used with other sedative or anaesthetic agents. Panting is sometimes seen after the administration of opioids (most often if the animal is not in pain) and is probably related to alteration of the thermoregulatory centre in the hypothalamus. This is most often seen with the administration of moderate to large doses of morphine or pethidine. Panting in dogs following administration of large doses of morphine or pethidine may also be due to a degree of histamine release and a degree of ensuing pulmonary oedema.

Animals that have sustained higher centre or brain-stem trauma will react unpredictably to drugs, particularly drugs that can depress the central nervous system, such as opioids, and thus the use of opioids in such cases should be carried out cautiously. If respiratory depression does occur, it can be reversed using an opiate antagonist, although this will also reverse any analgesia that has been provided. It may be preferable to use a specific respiratory stimulant such as doxapram, although this drug has a relatively short duration of action (10-20 min) and repeated administration may be required.

Opioids should also be used cautiously if respiratory depression is expected, as any further depression of respiration may become clinically relevant; however, pain (particularly thoracic or upper abdominal pain) can cause respiratory impairment, and the alleviation of pain usually more than compensates for any respiratory depression caused by the drug itself.

Cardiovascular effects
Most opioids have little effect. Morphine, fentanyl and alfentanil will cause bradycardia and hypotension if injected rapidly intravenously. Bradycardia is centrally mediated (vagal) and reversed by anticholinergics. Hypotension (resulting from histamine release or depression of the vasomotor centre) is avoided by slow intravenous administration or by using the intramuscular route. Venous tone tends to be reduced, thereby reducing preload. This effect can be beneficial in managing congestive heart failure. Pethidine causes histamine

release and thus hypotension if injected intravenously in the dog and to a lesser extent in the cat, and is contraindicated by this route. Pethidine has also been reported to exhibit a degree of myocardial depression, but this is probably not important clinically. Etorphine has pronounced effects: hypotension in the dog, and hypertension and tachycardia in the horse.

Gastro-intestinal effects

Following administration, a period of gastro-intestinal (GI) hypermotility with an increase in non-propulsive rhythmic contractions and an increase in smooth muscle tone including sphincter tone (including biliary and pancreatic ducts) can be seen; this is followed by a period of GI stasis.

Vomiting (activation of the chemoreceptor trigger zone) can be seen (particularly with morphine) and is often accompanied by defaecation. Vomiting is seen particularly with morphine-type drugs, and is a particular problem if such drugs are administered to 'pain free' animals. This must be borne in mind when designing 'pre-emptive' protocols.

The partial agonists such as buprenorphine are associated with less adverse effects on the GI tract. Pethidine has a spasmolytic action on the gut due to its anticholinergic action (pethidine was synthesised after work on atropine-like compounds), and does not cause spasm of biliary and pancreatic ducts. It is therefore indicated as an analgesic in cases of pancreatitis or biliary stasis, whereas use of other opioids in these circumstances is to be avoided.

Depression of the cough reflex

Drugs active at the μ- and κ-sites are effective antitussive agents. μ-Opioid receptors may inhibit antitussive activity. All opioids have a degree of antitussive activity by depressing the 'cough' centre in the medulla, but there is poor association between antitussive and analgesic properties of opioids. Codeine and butorphanol have antitussive activity at sub-analgesic doses.

Pruritis

Pruritis is sometimes seen after epidural or intrathecal administration of opioids, the itchy area being confined to the caudal dorsum of the animal. This is thought to be a result of low dose opioid enhancement of C-fibre activity.

Acute tolerance

Tolerance is the need for a bigger dose to achieve the same pharmacological effect. In clinical veterinary practice, the reason for needing to increase the dose is uniformly due to an increase in the pain. Acute tolerance has been shown to occur in the laboratory after the administration of large doses of opiates to pain-free animals. However, it also does not appear to be a problem in animals being administered pre-emptive analgesia [2]. Dependence is the need to continue drug administration after prior exposure to prevent the development of an abstinence syndrome. This does not appear to be a major problem in animals, or is not recognised.

Use of opioids in neonatal or aged animals, or animals with hepatic disease

Young age, old age or hepatic disease are not contraindications to the use of opioids; however, care should be exercised and lower doses used in such patients with reduced liver function because opioids are metabolised by hepatic enzymes and are often conjugated with glucuronic acid.

Ceiling effect with partial agonists / agonist-antagonist drugs

The use of partial agonists such as buprenorphine or agonist-antagonists such as butorphanol is believed to be associated with significant disadvantages compared to full μ-opioid agonists. As with much veterinary pharmacology, the original evidence for the actions of buprenorphine appear to have been extrapolated from human and laboratory studies. Buprenorphine has been shown to have a bell-shaped analgesic dose response curve in rats and mice. This means that beyond certain limits, increased doses of drug lead to a decreased analgesic action. In addition, buprenorphine, a partial agonist, has been shown in rats and mice to antagonise the analgesic action of pure μ-opioid agonists.

However, in these laboratory studies, antagonism of the analgesia produced by lower doses of buprenorphine occurred at doses 100 - 150 times those currently used in dogs (current dog doses are 10 - 20 µg/kg). At these doses, the respiratory depression effects and the enhanced gastro-intestinal motility induced by the lower doses of buprenorphine were also antagonised. In other analgesic tests (tail pressure test and writhing test), there was no antagonism of the analgesia even with the administration of doses corresponding to 2350-4700 times those currently used in dogs. Antagonism of morphine analgesia was demonstrated in rats in the tail flick latency test, but antagonism was not seen in rats in the tail pressure test.

It is these properties seen in experimental studies that have resulted in excessive caution in the clinical use of buprenorphine, with repeat doses denied to animals still in pain after buprenorphine administration. There has also been reluctance to use effective pure opioid agonists for essential pain relief in animals that have had buprenorphine premedication.

Single dose studies with buprenorphine at doses extrapolated from medical literature have demonstrated its efficacy as a perioperative analgesic in cats and dogs. The effects of multiple doses of buprenorphine and its effects on pure µ-agonist action clinically are being investigated at the moment. Evidence in sheep suggests that the bell-shaped dose response curve for analgesia may not be relevant to all species. Thus, further studies to elucidate the pharmacology of buprenorphine in dogs and cats are merited. This information should have a considerable impact on the welfare of clinical patients. A recent survey of UK veterinarians [3, 4] found that the prescription of analgesics to animals post-operatively was poor (for example, only 56% of bitches and 39% of cats undergoing ovariohysterectomy received any analgesics), and single doses of an analgesic were most often used. It also highlighted the side effects of opioids, and the fact that they are generally controlled drugs was a significant deterrent to their use. Buprenorphine is not a Schedule 2 controlled drug in the United Kingdom, and accurate guidelines on its clinical use would probably have considerable positive impact on the provision of analgesics to companion animals.

At the moment, it appears that buprenorphine can be used at higher than recommended doses, and more frequently, at least in the dog and the cat. Occasionally 'failures' are noted, and at such times, the sequential administration of pure μ-agonists appears to produce analgesia.

Notes on some of the more commonly used opioid drugs:

Morphine
Morphine is still the analgesic of choice for the most severe pain - there is no ceiling to its effect, so increasing the dose increases the analgesia. Following administration, the onset of action is not rapid; however its duration of action is longer than its plasma half-life would suggest. Morphine is metabolised by conjugation, and it is not surprising that its half-life is longer in the cat than in the dog (3 hours *versus* 60 minutes). At doses of 0.1-0.2 mg/kg given i.m. or s.c., morphine produces effective analgesia in cats for 6-8 hours without adverse excitatory side effects. Doses of 0.1-0.5 mg/kg can be used in dogs, but the duration of action is only about 1.5-3 hours.

Morphine can cause vomiting in dogs and cats (particularly those that are not experiencing pain) and is thus contraindicated following ocular surgery or gastric surgery.

Pethidine
This is a synthetic compound with an atropine-like structure. Like morphine, it is a μ-selective agonist, but unlike morphine it is devoid of adverse gastrointestinal effects. Its onset of action is more rapid than morphine, but its duration of action is relatively short. At a dose of 5-10 mg/kg i.m. it provides analgesia for 1.5-2 hours post-operatively in the cat, and it is used at a dose of 3-5 mg/kg in the dog, providing analgesia for up to 1.5 hours. If the subcutaneous route of administration is employed, then it is more difficult to achieve effective plasma concentrations of the drug, and a dose of 10-15 mg/kg should be used in cats and 5-10 mg/kg in dogs.

The clinical value of pethidine lies in its relative lack of unpleasant side effects and its excellent sedative properties. Its fast onset of action and its predictability makes it a very useful analgesic. When monitoring animals post-operatively its relatively short duration of action may not be such a drawback. Its atropine-like structure gives it spasmolytic properties, which makes it very useful following intestinal surgery and in cats with urolithiasis.

Methadone
Methadone is very similar to morphine. It is associated with less sedation than morphine, and vomiting is not seen so often. It is used at a dose of 0.1-0.5 mg/kg i.m. or i.v. in the dog and 0.1-0.3 mg/kg i.m. in the cat
The duration of action is approximately 2-3 hours in the dog and 3-5 hours in the cat at these doses.

Fentanyl
Fentanyl is a full agonist with a rapid onset of action (1 min), but short duration of action (15-20 minutes analgesia), making it impractical for long-term pain control. It is primarily used intra-operatively at doses of 1-4 µg/kg as required to augment the anaesthetic, or it can be used post-operatively as a short term measure to effect pain relief while longer acting opioids are given time to take effect. It has also been administered transdermally to good effect in some situations. Dose dependant respiratory depression can be seen.

Buprenorphine
Buprenorphine is a partial agonist at the µ-receptor. Thus, while low doses are analgesic, higher doses may theoretically be less effective - although the author believes that the clinical relevance of this is now in doubt (see above). Clinically it is probably very difficult to reach the 'ceiling', but the dose at which antagonism occurs in dogs and cats is not known. It has a slow onset of action, and is not equally effective against different types of pain. However, it does have a very long duration of action. These pharmacological properties have clinical implications. Firstly, the dose must be chosen carefully and top-up doses given only at 6-8 hour intervals (8-hour intervals in the cat). Secondly, the slow onset of action means that the drug must be given about 45 minutes before the analgesic effect is required. If animals are allowed to recover in pain before the drug has had an opportunity to be effective then it is less likely to be successful. Once buprenorphine

binds to the receptor it is very difficult to displace; thus, conventional antagonists cannot easily reverse its actions, nor can alternative opioid analgesic agents be used to top up analgesia. Buprenorphine should be reserved for less painful types of procedures, or those where other classes of analgesics are also being used. It can provide 4-6 hours analgesia in dogs (at 10-20 µg/kg) and 6-8 hours analgesia in the cat (at 20-40 µg/kg i/m).

Butorphanol

In addition to being a µ-partial agonist, butorphanol is an agonist on the kappa receptor. Like buprenorphine, its effect may reach a plateau or ceiling as the dose increases. This is certainly the case in the dog and cat where the optimal dose for visceral analgesia seems to be 0.2 mg/kg. Its efficacy against somatic pain is very poor at doses from 0.2-0.8 mg/kg. It has a very short elimination half-life and clinically appears to give only brief (30-40 min) analgesia post-operatively, with a relatively high number of 'failures'. Its effectiveness as a sedative and antitussive appear to be better than its analgesic potency in the cat and dog, and it should only be used for procedures expected to produce mild to moderate pain. It provides very effective sedation and this is often confused for effective analgesia.

Nalbuphine

Nalbuphine is an antagonist at the µ-receptor, an agonist at the delta receptor, and a partial agonist at the κ-receptor, and therefore its action is a mixture of agonist and antagonist activity. Rather than producing euphoria, it tends to cause dysphoria, but less so than the similar drug pentazocine. Like buprenorphine, its effect may reach a plateau or ceiling as the dose increases. It is said to have minimal sedative effects and minimal effects on respiration. At doses of 0.05-0.1 mg/kg, given i.m. or i.v., it can provide effective analgesia for up to 2 hours. It can be associated with pain upon injection.

Naloxone and naltrexone

Naloxone and naltrexone are antagonists used to reverse the effects of agonists and agonist-antagonists. These drugs attach competitively to all opioid receptors and displace the opioid drug. Naloxone has a short duration of action (30-60 minutes) and therefore repeat doses of naloxone are often necessary.

Local anaesthetics

Local anaesthetics block action potential transmission along nerve fibres. The most widely used drugs in this class are lignocaine and bupivacaine. Others include cocaine, procaine, amethocaine, mepivacaine and prilocaine. The mechanism of action is one of stabilisation of the cell membrane. The drugs act by preventing the depolarization-induced transient opening of the voltage-dependent Na^+ conducting channels in the axonal membrane, thus preventing the generation of the spike component of the action potential. Local anaesthetics are ideal as pre-emptive analgesics as they potentially block all nociceptive information travelling in the target nerve, and because of this complete block, they can decrease the requirement for general anaesthetic agents. Recovery from local anaesthesia occurs when the local concentration of the drug falls, following its absorption from its site of administration and action. It is at this time that these drugs may produce their toxic effects if the rate of absorption is fast enough to exceed the rate of biotransformation. Local anaesthetics are often combined with adrenaline (1:100,000 or 1:200,000 dilutions). Adrenaline causes vasoconstriction and prolongs the action of the drug, and diminishes the rate of absorption. Local anaesthetic without adrenaline should be used in high-risk patients to avoid any possible cardiac stimulation and also when performing 'blocks' of appendages to avoid any compromise to the blood supply to the area. More usually however, toxicity results from the direct uncontrolled injection of the drug into the systemic circulation. Local anaesthetics can cause hypotension, dysrythmias, e.g. atrioventricular block, and central nervous system depression and then seizures. With these drugs, sedation is seen first, then agitation, restlessness, vomiting and then seizure activity and finally complete CNS depression. Many of the local anaesthetics (e.g. bupivacaine and lignocaine) are toxic to tissues, but this is probably of little clinical relevance unless concurrent factors delay healing. Bupivacaine dissociates quite slowly from sodium channels and cardiotoxic effects are more marked. Toxic doses are 20 mg/kg for lignocaine and 4 mg/kg for bupivacaine, given intravenously, and so safe maximum doses are 4 mg/kg lignocaine and 1-2 mg/kg bupivicaine. Care needs to be exercised when dosing cats and small dogs with local anaesthetics because they are at greater risk of overdose. Lignocaine has a rapid onset (onset 1-2 minutes) and short duration (1.5-2 hours) of action. Bupivacaine has a slower onset of action (5-10 minutes) but much longer duration of action (4-6 hours).

Local anaesthetic techniques are not difficult to perform after some practice, so that the drugs block the transmission of impulses between the surgical site and the CNS. Local anaesthetics have been administered in small doses systemically intravenously for post-operative pain and for cancer pain in humans, but so far there are no reports of this method of administration to treat pain in animals.

Local anaesthetics may be employed in several ways:

- topically
Local anaesthetic can be deposited around exposed nerves during surgery, for example, during forelimb amputations the nerves of the brachial plexus can be bathed in local anaesthetic prior to transection. Although surgery has started, the amount of nociceptive information generated by the transection of a nerve is considerable, and prior blocking of the nerve markedly decreases the associated post-operative pain.

Exposed nasal turbinate mucosa can be desensitised using local anaesthetic spray, and local anaesthetic gels can be spread on the rectum following rectal or peri-rectal surgery to provide analgesia and decrease tenesmus.

- by local tissue infiltration
This can be carried out near to the surgical site or along the line of incision through cutaneous tissues, either prior to incision or at the end of surgery prior to wound closure.

- by tissue infiltration to block a region
Local anaesthetic can be injected around a distal limb or around the base of a digit prior to distal limb surgery or amputation respectively. A detailed knowledge of the anatomy of the area is not required. When blocking extremities with such 'ring blocks', local anaesthetic *without* adrenaline should be used to prevent tissue ischaemia as a result of the constrictive effect of adrenaline on local

blood vessels. Another example of a regional block is the inverted L block used in cattle to block the paravertebral nerves to the abdominal wall.

- intravenous regional anaesthesia
Local anaesthetics can be administered into a distal vein of a limb with a tourniquet applied proximally in order to produce analgesia of the area below the tourniquet prior to carrying out digit amputation or other distal limb surgery.

- by tissue infiltration to block specific nerves
If the anatomy of the area is known, local anaesthetic can be injected accurately to block the sensory nerves carrying pain impulses from the surgical field. For example, intercostal nerve blocks prior to lateral thoracotomy, distal intercostal nerve block prior to or following sternotomy, maxillary and mandibular alveolar nerve blocks, brachial plexus block in small animals, pudendal nerve block in cattle and individual nerve blocks to the distal limb in horses.

- by instillation into a cavity
Local anaesthetic can be flushed into the thoracic cavity through a thoracotomy tube to provide analgesia following thoracotomy. Local anaesthetic can also be instilled into a pleural catheter or an over-the-needle catheter instead of the chest drain. Instillation of local anaesthetic into the abdomen can be very effective for upper abdominal pain, but is not very effective for general abdominal pain.

Doses of 0.5 mg/kg bupivacaine or 1.0 mg/kg lignocaine can be instilled into joints of dogs following surgery once the joint has been effectively sealed [5]. This method is extremely simple and provides very effective and safe post-operative analgesia after stifle and shoulder arthrotomies.

- by extradural or spinal administration
Local anaesthetics can be administered pre-operatively into the intradural or sub-arachnoid ('spinal') spaces, either alone or in combination with opioid or alpha-adrenergic agonists. Similar combinations can also be used in the epidural space.

NSAIDs

Until relatively recently, the drugs available were less effective than opioids for severe pain, but the picture has changed with the new generation of NSAIDs now on the market. Many of the classical NSAIDs are very toxic, especially in the cat, which is unable to conjugate and eliminate these drugs effectively due to a deficiency of bilirubin-glucuronoside glucuronosyltransferase enzyme.

NSAIDs have been defined as those substances other than steroids that suppress one or more components of the inflammatory process. The group of compounds is restricted to those substances that act by inhibiting components of the enzyme system in the metabolism of arachidonic acid and the formation of eicosanoids. Eicosanoids include the prostanoids (prostaglandins; prostacyclin, PGI_2; thromboxane, TXA_2) and leukotrienes.

However, the NSAIDs are a heterogeneous group of compounds, often chemically unrelated, and further research over the years has shown the situation with respect to some of the NSAIDs to be far more complex and poorly understood.

Prostanoids are unsaturated fatty acid compounds derived from 20-carbon essential fatty acids, the most important precursor being arachidonic acid. They function for the most part as local hormones, with their biological activity exerted primarily at their site of synthesis, as their half-life is very short. The synthesis and release of prostanoids is influenced by various physiological stimuli including peptide hormones (angiotensin II, vasopressin), catecholamines and mechanical trauma. The biological effects of the prostanoids are diverse and include smooth muscle contraction, vasodilatation, platelet aggregation and disaggregation, gastrointestinal secretion, release of other hormones, central nervous system stimulation and depression and mediation of the inflammatory response.

Prostaglandins (particularly PGE_2 and PGI_2) play a role in the production of a noxious stimulus at the periphery (inflammatory pain) by sensitising receptors on afferent nerve endings to the actions of bradykinin and histamine, other compounds released in the inflammatory process. Prostaglandins, by virtue of their actions in the central nervous system, also play an important part in facilitating the transmission of 'painful' stimuli (noxious stimuli) that are travelling into and through the spinal cord to higher centres. This occurs particularly during prolonged or severe post-operative pain and in chronic pain. Thus, drugs inhibiting the production of prostaglandins by the inhibition of cyclo-oxygenase (COX) will produce analgesic effects by their actions both at the periphery and centrally.

Side effects of NSAIDs

However, the toxicity of NSAIDs is also related to their inhibition of prostaglandin production, and disruption of the processes they participate in, resulting principally in various degrees of renal function impairment and gastrointestinal irritation and ulceration. The incidence of side effects is significant, and although the clinical incidence in animals is not documented, in human medicine in the US, long-term use of NSAIDs causes stomach ulcers so severe that they kill about 7000 people a year. Other adverse effects seen in animals are blood dyscrasias (e.g. with phenylbutazone), liver damage and worsening cardiac failure due to water retention. It is therefore most important to consider the efficacy : toxicity ratio for any particular NSAID prior to use in any particular species.

The kidney is extremely active in the synthesis and metabolism of prostaglandins, where they participate in autoregulation of renal blood flow and glomerular filtration, modulation of renin release, tubular ion transport and water metabolism. In the kidney, locally produced prostaglandins are continually active in maintaining afferent arteriolar dilation, and at times of volume depletion, i.e. relative or absolute hypovolaemia (such as occurs with administration of most anaesthetic agents, blood loss, peritonitis, cardiac failure, septic shock or endotoxaemia) these prostaglandins assume a very important role in the maintenance of normal renal haemodynamics. If, under such circumstances, the production of these prostaglandins is inhibited, that is, steroids or classical NSAIDs are administered at times of volume depletion, renal hypoperfusion will result, and a degree of renal failure may occur.

The ulcerogenicity of NSAIDs is correlated to their ability to inhibit cyclo-oxygenase (COX). PGE$_2$ and PGI$_2$ promote the secretion of protective mucus along the intestinal tract, and play a role in the modulation of the production of gastric acid. Inhibition of the production of these prostaglandins when steroids or classical NSAIDs are administered, can result in various degrees of gastro-intestinal irritation and ulceration.

NSAIDs inhibit proteoglycan synthesis, and proteoglycan synthesis is greatly increased and therefore more severely affected in osteoarthritis. Some manufacturers claim that different NSAIDs have different properties in this respect. It is unlikely that any of the currently available NSAIDs have a chondroprotective effect; however, recent work has suggested that meloxicam and carprofen may have a chondroneutral effect at therapeutic doses, that is, they may not have an adverse effect on cartilage metabolism.

COX-1 and COX-2

New impetus to the field of analgesia and inflammation research was provided by the finding that the cyclo-oxygenase enzyme (COX) exists in (at least) two different forms. It was found that COX activity was stimulated by bacterial endotoxin and that this increase in activity was due to the *de novo* synthesis of new COX protein. Shortly after this, the inducible COX protein was characterised as a distinct isoform of cyclo-oxygenase (COX-2) and shown to be coded by a different gene from that producing the constitutive enzyme, renamed COX-1. Thus there are now known to be two types of cyclo-oxygenase enzyme, one producing 'essential prostaglandins' on a minute-to-minute basis, and another which becomes activated as a result of tissue trauma and results in the production of 'inflammatory or pain mediating prostaglandins'. Inducible COX (COX-2) has now been identified in most cell types involved in inflammation, and there is evidence that COX-2 iso-enzyme might be responsible for the production of prostaglandins at inflammatory sites and thus be the relevant target for the therapeutic effects of NSAIDs. The inhibition of the constitutive enzyme, COX-1, and thus a decrease in the production of 'essential prostaglandins' is considered to be responsible for the gastric and renal toxic side effects as well as the anti-thrombotic activity of NSAIDs.

COX-1 is constitutively expressed in most tissues, functioning to synthesise prostaglandins which regulate normal cellular function - it has been termed the 'cellular housekeeping' enzyme. The inhibition of COX-1 leads to the well-known toxic side effects of NSAIDs - gastric ulceration and renal toxicity. COX-2 is not found in resting cells in any significant amounts, but its expression is increased dramatically in inflammatory states - COX-2 is part of the body's 'crisis intervention system'. Unfortunately, most existing NSAIDs block not only the action of COX-2, but also the action of COX-1, leaving the body short of 'housekeeping' prostaglandins. The discovery of COX-2 opened the door to finding drugs that would block only the action of this enzyme, so reducing pain and inflammation, while leaving the housekeeping functions of COX-1 untouched. However, recently, the situation has become less clear cut, with the finding that COX-2 may be expressed 'constitutively' in some cells or organs, and be essential for normal function.

A series of NSAIDs have been tested for their relative activities against COX-1 and COX-2 in whole cell preparations, and tables of activity ratios have been constructed. The IC_{50} (μM) ratios COX-2/COX-1 that are published refer to the ratios of the concentration of the drug that causes 50% inhibition of each iso-enzyme in the test system used. Thus, a ratio of less than 1.00 suggests a preferential activity of the drug against COX-2, i.e. a smaller concentration of drug is required to inhibit COX-2 than is required to inhibit COX-1. The values reported appear to vary widely from study to study depending on whether the drugs have been tested against cells from the target species or not; whether or not the COX-1 and COX-2 assays have been carried out using the same or different cell types; and the exact conditions under which the experiment has been performed. As yet there does not appear to be any 'standard' test system, nor any test system from which the results can be used to predict what will happen clinically. To add confusion to the area, some workers report COX-1/COX-2 ratios where a value of less than 1.00 suggests a preferential inhibition by the drug of COX-1, and a ratio of greater than 1.00 suggests preferential inhibition of COX-2. This article will consider the more widely used COX-2/COX-1 ratio.

Some of the reported ratios for the newer NSAIDs licensed for use in the dog are (data taken from [6-9] and unpublished data):

Drug	Ratio COX-2 / COX-1
Meloxicam	0.08-0.8
Carprofen	0.01-1.0
Ketoprofen	5.0
Tolfenamic acid	0.1-16.7

It has been realised however, that interpretation and extrapolation of data from different studies is greatly hampered by the variability in the test systems used in individual studies. A qualitative comparison of the COX-2/COX-1 ratios of different NSAIDs can only be made within one experimental set-up and test system.

As a comparison, in the test systems used, piroxicam (ratio of 250), Aspirin (ratio of 166) and indomethacin (ratio of 60) showed the worst COX-2/COX-1 ratios, i.e. they were very much more selective for COX-1 than for COX-2. These drugs are well known for their propensity to cause gastric ulceration. From the above table, meloxicam and carprofen would appear to have the most favourable COX-2/COX-1 ratios, i.e. they produce selective inhibition of COX-2, followed by ketoprofen and then tolfenamic acid. Experimentally, drugs that are more selective towards COX-2 inhibition seem to have a high gastric tolerance and high renal tolerance.

Small structural alterations in a compound have been shown to significantly alter the selectivity of the compound for COX-2 over COX-1, and there are now a number of compounds being tested for the human market that show *over 1000-fold activity against COX-2 than for COX-1* (i.e. a ratio of 0.001), and as such, also potentially have much less toxicity at the gastric mucosa and at the kidney under experimental conditions. Such *truly selective* COX-2 inhibitors are not available for the human market yet, and are unlikely to be available for the veterinary market for some time.

However, an important aspect to consider is the overall total inhibition of cox-1 and thus likelihood of side effects, that is, the efficacy: toxicity ratio. All the NSAIDs that have been tested in dogs, with the exception of carprofen, have been shown to significantly inhibit the production of thromboxane B_2 by platelets. This assay is used to predict the degree of cyclo-oxygenase (cox-1) inhibition that will take place in the target species administered a therapeutic dose of the drug. Thus, although a compound may be a preferential cox-2 inhibitor, if it still has significant cox-1 inhibition, it will still be likely to produce side effects.

The peri-operative use of NSIADs

During anaesthesia and surgery, patients may suffer relative or absolute hypovolaemia (as a result of pre-existing shock or because of blood loss during surgery or as a result of the hypotensive nature of the anaesthetic agents) and the kidney becomes reliant on locally produced prostaglandins to maintain normal renal perfusion.

Of the NSAIDs currently available for use in small animals, carprofen is the only one considered to be safe for pre- or peri-operative administration [10, 11], although recent unpublished work has also shown that meloxicam is safe in this respect. In the case of carprofen, this is probably due to its reduced effect on the production of prostaglandins (its mechanism of action is unknown), and its postulated preferential inhibition of cox-2, and in the case of meloxicam is probably due to its consistent preferential inhibition of cox-2. This serves to underline the fact that the NSAIDs are a heterogeneous group of compounds, and should not all be thought of as 'clones' of Aspirin. Two studies have examined the effect of administering a NSAID (carprofen) prior to surgery *versus* after surgery, and found it to be more effective if administered prior to surgery [10, 11].

Animals that are being medicated with NSAIDs orally and need to undergo anaesthesia and surgery should either have the NSAID medication discontinued 36 hours prior to the procedure, or be maintained on high enough rates of fluid administration under anaesthesia to maintain normal blood pressure, and fluid administration should be continued into the post-operative period until the cardiovascular system is not any longer under the effect of residual levels of anaesthetic agents.

Notes on the individual NSAIDs:

Acetylsalicylic acid (Aspirin)

This causes gastric irritation in cats and dogs, aplastic anaemia and hepatoxicity in cats, as its half-life is so long (40 hours in cats) that cumulation will occur. Until recently, it was the most extensively used anti-inflammatory agent in the USA, despite the fact that adverse effects are common after its use, with dose dependant epithelial damage and haemorrhages developing within 4 hours of its administration orally. This extensive use was probably due to the fact that there were few other NSAIDs available, and it was accepted that side effects would be seen. Buffered or enteric coated Aspirin is often recommended to decrease the risk of GI haemorrhage and ulceration; such recommendations are inferred from advertisements for human beings, and there is no evidence to support such claims in dogs. Fixed dose preparations of codeine and Aspirin are available, but at high doses, the toxic side effects of Aspirin limit the analgesic effects of codeine.

Phenylbutazone

This drug is particularly toxic in the cat, and to a lesser extent in the dog. It has particularly been associated with blood dyscrasias, hepatopathy and nephropathy, gastro-intestinal haemorrhage, and occasionally irreversible bone marrow suppression.

Flunixin meglumine

This drug is extremely potent as an analgesic but can also cause severe gastro-intestinal and renal damage. It has a shorter half-life in the cat than the dog, but nevertheless should be used with extreme caution in either species, particularly around the time of anaesthesia and surgery, and certainly should not be used pre-operatively. It has been shown to increase survival of dogs in models of septic shock in the dog, although this has never been followed up clinically. It is used quite extensively for endotoxaemia in the horse.

Ketoprofen

Ketoprofen is a powerful inhibitor of both cyclo-oxygenase and lipo-oxygenase enzymes, and inhibits bradykinin. It is, therefore, a very effective anti-inflammatory agent and a good analgesic, but because of its inhibition of prostaglandin production, it should not be used pre-operatively, but rather post-operatively in the recovery phase.

Tolfenamic acid

Tolfenamic acid is a powerful inhibitor of cyclo-oxygenase, and the comments above on ketoprofen apply to tolfenamic acid.

Vedaprofen

Vedaprofen is a powerful inhibitor of cyclo-oxygenase, and the comments above on ketoprofen and tolfenamic acid apply also to vedaprofen.

Meloxicam

Meloxicam is a powerful inhibitor of prostaglandin production and is a very effective analgesic. It is marketed as a preferential COX-2 inhibitor and, indeed, studies have consistently shown it to be a preferential COX-2 inhibitor. Trials in humans have shown it to be very safe in terms of gastro-intestinal toxicity, and studies have shown it to be well tolerated in dogs and cats, although gastro-intestinal side effects seem to be the most likely side effects to be seen. Meloxicam has recently been shown to be safe for administration pre-operatively to dogs. However, it is possible to decrease the dose substantially after initiating a course, whilst maintaining efficacy. Once daily dosing is all that seems to be required initially, and after the first 5 days, the dosing interval can be increased up to 2 or 3 days in some dogs. Meloxicam seems to be particularly useful for animals suffering joint pain as a result of an old injury such as a fracture.

Carprofen

Carprofen, despite being an excellent anti-inflammatory and potent analgesic agent, is postulated to have relatively little effect on prostaglandin production. It seems to be tolerated extremely well with very few side effects being reported. In the UK, the injectable form has undergone extensive use clinically pre-operatively with good effect and no reported side effects in cats and dogs. Investigative studies have shown it to be very effective and safe in dogs, both as a peri-operative analgesic given prior to the surgery, and also in long term administration to dogs, and for cats as a peri-operative analgesic. A few isolated cases of idiosyncratic hepatocellular necrosis have been reported in dogs.

Alpha2-adrenoceptor agonists

All the adrenoceptor agonists (e.g. medetomidine, detomidine, xylazine, romifidine) are potent analgesic agents, acting by binding to alpha2-receptors in the brain and spinal cord. There are at least 3 different subtypes of alpha2-adrenoceptor receptors; they are present in many tissues, although their distribution varies amongst species. Alpha2-adrenoceptor agonists have their actions mediated via these receptors, and possibly also imidazole receptors. Central actions include analgesia, sedation and hypnosis, and peripheral actions include reduced motility of the gastro-intestinal tract, platelet aggregation, a decrease in insulin secretion (thus hyperglycaemic effects), and a reduction in ACTH and also ADH (leading to diuresis). Alpha2-agonists cause a centrally mediated reduction in sympathetic drive and a vagally mediated bradycardia, and peripherally cause vasoconstriction resulting in hypertension. In low doses, central actions, such as vasodilatation, predominate, and so the overall effect is dose dependant and varies from drug to drug.

Alpha2-agonists have marked analgesic actions. However, in veterinary medicine, the drugs are used mainly for their sedative effects. If an antagonist (e.g. atipamezole) is used to reverse the effects of the drug, the analgesic effect is also reversed. Alpha2-adrenoceptor agonists have been used epidurally to good effect, with medetomidine producing better analgesia in the cat than in the dog. Xylazine has been successfully used epidurally to provide analgesia in dogs (at 0.25-0.75 mg/kg) and also horses (0.25 mg/kg). The chance of seeing side effects following epidural alpha adrenoceptor agonist in horses is reported to be less with xylazine than detomidine. Side effects can be seen following epidurally administered medetomidine (0.015 mg/kg) in dogs, such as vomiting and bradycardia, due to systemic spread. Xylazine is used extensively in cattle to provide analgesia, and detomidine and romifidine in horses. Romifidine is suggested to be associated with less ataxia than detomidine. The concurrent sedative effects seen with their use usually limit the post-operative use of these drugs.

Dissociative agents

Excitatory amino acids (EAAs) play an important role in spinal nociceptive processing (see previous chapter). Glutamate is the most important endogenous EAA, and can act on either ionotropic receptors (including the NMDA receptor) and metabotropic receptors. The NMDA receptor, together with the neurokinin receptors 1 and 2, plays a key role in central sensitisation, which is probably the key to persistent and chronic pain states. Antagonism of the NMDA receptor experimentally often results in analgesia in such situations of facilitated spinal nociceptive processing.

Ketamine is a non-competitive NMDA antagonist. Ketamine appears to be effective in preventing central sensitisation in certain situations. It is a good analgesic against ischaemic and somatic pain, although it has a relatively short duration of action (30 minutes) at low doses (0.1-0.2 mg/kg). Higher doses will provide longer duration of analgesia, but will induce dissociative anaesthesia. It is the hallucinatory and other disturbances that limit the usefulness of ketamine as an analgesic. There is some evidence that ketamine and other NMDA antagonists may act synergistically with opioids in providing analgesia, adding more weight to the argument for 'multi-modal' analgesia (see later).

Inhalational agents

With the exception of nitrous oxide, the inhalational agents should be considered as not providing any significant analgesia. Nitrous oxide is a useful analgesic in man, and is reported to be only slightly less effective in the dog as an analgesic. It should be used at a concentration of at least 50% to provide analgesia. The mechanism of action is not known, and it is contraindicated in situations where further accumulation of gas in an already existing pocket of gas would be detrimental, e.g. gastric dilatation prior to effective decompression.

Benzodiazepines

These may have some analgesic activity, but the main beneficial effect in pain therapy is to cause muscle relaxation (at a level of internuncial neurones in the spinal cord) and thus decreasing the amount of nociceptive information going into the spinal cord from spastic muscles. Thus very useful in spinal surgery cases or any cases where muscle spasm is producing a component of the pain.

Routes of administration of analgesics

Two clinical issues sometimes become confused in discussions of alternative routes of administration of analgesics. The first is clinical necessity - some patients may have to have medication administered by particular routes. The second is the potential of new routes of analgesic administration to provide better analgesia and / or fewer side effects. Often these alternative routes (e.g. epidural) do provide longer lasting or better analgesia, but systemic absorption can and does occur, and the risk of seeing systemic side effects still exists. Obviously, there is also often a particular risk or side effect associated with administration of the analgesic by a 'novel' route, and the choice of which route to use in any particular animal must be made on an individual basis. General notes are given in Table 3.

Transdermal route

Transdermal patches consisting of an adhesive layer, a release membrane that controls the delivery of the drug, a drug reservoir and a protective backing layer have been used to administer fentanyl. The drug is administered in a slow continuous manner, potentially avoiding the problems of over and underdosing associated with bolus administration. Fentanyl has a low molecular weight and high lipid solubility, making it an ideal drug for transdermal delivery. It has been shown to be an effective, well-tolerated, long-lasting and relatively inexpensive means of providing post-operative analgesia. The patches are available in four sizes (25, 50, 75 and 100 μg/h) and an appropriate patch should be chosen on the basis of the size of the dog to provide 2-4 μg/kg/h. After application, 12-24 hours are required in the canine patient to reach effective plasma concentrations and these are maintained for 72 hours. They are probably best used if placed on the patient 24 hours prior to surgery, and other classes of analgesics

Table 3

General notes on routes of administration of analgesics

Route	Notes
Intravenous	As with any drug, always inject slowly – best route for opioids, unless otherwise indicated, e.g. pethidine Good for some NSAIDs – but action seems somewhat shorter. Often used to administer carprofen pre-operatively.
Intramuscular	Not necessarily 'safer' than intravenous, only lower plasma concentrations reached. Absorption from intramuscular sites is very variable. In dogs and cats, triceps and lumbar muscles are generally more predictably perfused than quadriceps muscles.
Subcutaneous	Generally ineffective for opioids (unless much higher doses used) Seems very effective for some NSAIDs due to high bioavailability from this site Effective for ketamine (low dose infusions used s.c. or i.m. in humans to control chronic pain)
Oral	NSAIDs for control of chronic pain and post-op. follow-up analgesia Opioids may be used by this route more in the future for the control of chronic pain
Local infiltration/ application	Local anaesthetics
Transdermal	NSAID gels (human preparations) may be used more in the future Fentanyl patches
Intra-articular	Local anaesthetics and opioids can be used by this route to produce effective analgesia
Epidural / spinal	Opioids, local anaesthetics and alpha adrenergic agonists can be used effectively by this route NSAIDs and ketamine may be used more in the future

used to augment analgesia pre- and post-operatively. Problems have been seen with dispensing fentanyl in this form as it can be reconstituted from the patch and subsequently abused. It is likely such patches will only be used for the peri-operative or long-term management of pain in hospitalised patients.

Epidural (outside the inner layer of dura)

Opioids, local anaesthetics and alpha adrenoceptor agonists can be used effectively by this route. These drugs can be administered either as single injections, as multiple injections with needles or an implanted catheter, or as a continuous infusion through an implanted catheter. In the future, more use is likely to be made of epidural (or spinal) administration of such drugs, and possibly NSAIDs and ketamine. Lower doses than are used systemically can be used, and although systemic absorption can occur, the systemic side effects normally seen with the drugs are generally less, and the duration of analgesia longer (a dose of 0.1 mg/kg morphine can provide analgesia for up to 20 hours). Preservative-free formulations of the drugs should be used to avoid adverse effects on the spinal cord.

Morphine, oxymorphone, fentanyl and buprenorphine are most commonly used. Specific side effects associated with the epidural use of opioids are urinary retention (more often seen after repeated injections) and localised hyperaesthesia or pruritis. If local anaesthetics such as bupivacaine and lignocaine are used, loss of motor function caudally and possibly hypotension (due to pooling of blood in the splanchnic circulation following blockade of the sympathetic outflow) can occur. In dogs, the dural sac usually ends cranial to the lumbosacral space, but it rarely does in cats, and in cats the subdural space is often entered. If this occurs in either dogs or cats, the suggested doses should be decreased by 50%.

Opioids can be combined with local anaesthetics or alpha adrenoceptor agonists. These combinations can provide very long periods of analgesia - the combined effect is generally supra-additive - up to 24 hours. Epidural catheters can be placed to provide a means of administering further doses of analgesics post-operatively; however, it is the author's opinion that this is unnecessarily complex, and that excellent pre- and peri-operative analgesia can be provided by combinations of 'one shot' epidurals and NSAID therapy.

Intra-articular analgesia

Following arthrotomies, analgesics can be placed into the joint to provide effective and safe analgesia. Theoretically, local anaesthetics will block the sensory nerves carrying information from the joint and opioids bind to peripheral opioid receptors to produce analgesia. At the moment, it is unclear whether the activity of analgesics instilled into a joint is due solely due to the local effects or due to systemic effects after absorption from the joint, or due to a combination of the two. However, clinically, it appears that the administration of analgesics by this route is associated with fewer side effects than when the drug is administered systemically. The doses used are at the low end of the suggested doses for systemic administration (e.g. 0.1 mg/kg morphine; 0.5-1 mg/kg bupivacaine). The effect on cartilage and on the process of osteoarthritic disease is unknown, but clinically there does not appear to be a problem.

Pharmacological considerations when applying pre-emptive analgesia in surgical cases

Clinical pain is a combination of central hypersensitivity and peripheral hypersensitivity. Pre-emptive analgesic drug administration (that is, the administration of analgesics before the painful stimulus occurs) protects the dorsal horn neurones from the sensitising effect of the initial noxious stimulus (local anaesthetic or opioid administration) and reduces the severity of the inflammatory response and changes in the CNS (NSAID administration). This has been found both experimentally and clinically in animals for opioids and NSAIDs, and probably exists for alpha2-adrenoceptor agonists, local anaesthetics and ketamine. These strategies will prevent or markedly attenuate the development of post-operative hyperalgesia. However, the use of only one class of analgesic, even prior to surgery, is unlikely to provide effective analgesia in most instances (see below). Also, the clinician should attempt to match the degree of expected trauma from surgery with the doses and the duration of action of analgesics used.

Once the anaesthetic agents and protocol have been decided on, consideration should then be given to what analgesics are required in the light of what anaesthetics have been chosen, remembering that some anaesthetics provide analgesia as well (ketamine, alpha2-adrenoceptor agonists) whereas the majority do not (thiopentone, propofol, inhalant anaesthetics).

When considering an opioid dose and drug,
- *a pure μ-agonist should be chosen for potentially severe pain;*
- *an analgesic dose should be chosen, given at the correct time prior to surgery, either combined with the sedative (e.g. phenothiazine), or given separately to optimise its effectiveness;*
- *top-up doses should be planned if the single pre-operative dose is unlikely to last beyond the duration of surgery;*

When considering a NSAID for peri-operative use:
- *the clinician should consider if there are there any contraindications to the use of a NSAID in the particular case, such as concurrent steroid or NSAID therapy, pre-existing renal disease or pre-existing gastro-intestinal ulceration?*
- *the clinician should determine if the drug chosen is safe to be used prior to anaesthesia, or is it best given after recovery from anaesthesia?*

Consideration should also be made of any other analgesic drugs or regimens that could be used to augment analgesia in the particular case, e.g. local anaesthetics, ketamine, diazepam post-operatively.

The complexity of pain transmission and 'multi-modal' therapy

As more has become known about pain transmission over the last few years, it has become obvious that pain transmission involves a multiplicity of pathways and a multiplicity of mechanisms and transmitter systems. It is therefore unlikely that a single class of analgesic, whatever the dose, is likely to provide complete analgesia. This is confirmed by clinical experience. Much more effective is the combination of two or more classes of analgesics, e.g. opioids and

NSAIDS. The effect from these drugs is often supra-additive, and smaller doses of the individual drugs can be used, thus decreasing the likelihood of side effects from any one drug. So-called 'multi-modal' therapy is now recommended in clinical practice.

References

1 Joel E, Arndts F. Beitrange zur pharmakologie der korperstellung und der labyrinthreflexe.XIX. Mitteilung: Morphin. Arch. ges. Physio 1925:280-3.

2 Lascelles BDX, Cripps PJ, Jones A, Waterman-Pearson AE. Post-operative central hypersensitvity and pain: the pre-emptive value of pethidine for ovariohysterectomy. Pain 1997;73:461-71.

3 Capner CA, Lascelles BDX, Waterman-Peason AE. A survey of current British veterinary attitudes to peri-operative analgesia for dogs. Vet Rec 1999;145:95-9.

4 Lascelles BDX, Capner CA, Waterman-Peason AE. A survey of current British veterinary attitudes to peri-operative analgesia for cats and small mammals. Vet Rec 1999; *in press.*

5 Sammarco JL, Conzemius MG, Perkowski SZ, Weinstein MJ, Gregor TP, Smith GK. Postoperative analgesia for stifle surgery: A comparison of intra-articular bupivacaine, morphine, or saline. Vet Surg 1996;25:59-69.

6 Vane JR, Botting RM. New insights into the mode of action of anti-inflammatory drugs. Inflam Res 1995;44:1-10.

7 Battistini B, Botting R, Bakhle YS. COX-1 and COX-2: Toward the development of more selective NSAIDS. Drug News Perspect 1994; 7:501-12.

8 Ricketts AP, Lundy KM, Seibel SB. Evaluation of selective inhibition of canine cyclooxygenase 1 and 2 by carprofen and other nonsteroidal anti-inflammatory drugs. Am J Vet Res 1998;59:1441-6.

9 Kay-Mugford P, Conlon P, LaMarre J. In vitro evaluation of nonsteroidal antiinflammatory drugs for use in the dog. Am J Vet Res 1999; *in press.*

10 Lascelles BDX, Cripps PJ, Jones A, Waterman-Pearson AE. Efficacy and kinetics of carprofen, administered preoperatively or postoperatively, for the prevention of pain in dogs undergoing ovariohysterectomy Veterinary Surgery 1998;27:568-82.

11 Welsh EM, Nolan AM, Reid J. Beneficial effects of administering carprofen before surgery in dogs. Veterinary Record 1997; 141:251-3.

7

PRACTICAL ANALGESIC TREATMENT IN CANINE PATIENTS

Ludo J. Hellebrekers, DVM, PhD, DipECVA,
Faculty of Veterinary Medicine, Utrecht University,
Utrecht, The Netherlands

Introduction

When considering the physiology of pain it immediately becomes clear that it is of utmost importance to try to prevent pain from occurring, rather then attempting treatment once the pain is present. When effective prevention of pain is being targeted, the development of peripheral and/or central sensitisation does not occur, making the pain (control) easier to manage. It is obvious that this preventative action will not at all times be accomplished (i.e. in trauma cases) explaining why under such circumstances an effective pain control may only be partially achieved.

Prevention of the development of pain is not only a matter of a timely pre-anaesthetic administration of an analgesic, but also includes per- and post-surgery analgesic treatment. Treatment schedules with inadequate doses, too long dosing intervals or those insufficiently prolonged, will severely impair overall effectiveness of the analgesic treatment.

Although the insight in pain physiology clearly dictates a timely initiation of pain therapy, the discussion about whether or not to start pain therapy usually evolves around the problem of recognition of pain (symptoms) in our canine patients. The literature clearly shows that, under circumstances of close and detailed observation and scoring of pre-determined, well-defined behavioural elements, pain can be detected and its intensity estimated (see for further details Chapter 4).

Under conditions of veterinary practice, the observation will be hampered by all kinds of confounding influences, time constraints will limit the duration of observation, and overall conditions are such that an accurate estimation of the patient's pain will not be achieved.

A more practical approach is laid down in the *Principle of Analogy*, which states that those stimuli that are known to be painful in humans are to be considered painful in animals as well. This leads to a categorisation of procedures based upon the 'level of invasiveness', i.e. the severity of the (surgical) procedure, which subsequently dictates the relative weight or necessity of installing analgesic therapy. Veterinarians will need to consider the fact, for which clear support can be found in the literature, that the training in veterinary medicine does not automatically make them suited for assessing animal behaviour, let alone pain behaviour.

High-quality behavioural evaluation in animal patients potentially experiencing pain, requires more a specific theoretical and practical experience than is usually present, necessitates a distinctly systematic approach and will involve investing more time than is normally available during an average consultation.

As a consequence, veterinarians, in general, would be wise to refrain from basing their clinical practice on what they do or do not (perceive to) detect regarding behavioural signs of pain, and adopt the *Principle of Analogy* for their patients instead.

General therapeutic options for canine analgesic therapy

Especially in cases of elective surgical intervention, the importance of an adequate analgesic component in the premedication cannot be overestimated. Certainly, adequacy of analgesia during surgery must be ensured, but depending on the duration and level of invasiveness of the intervention, the analgesic administered pre-surgically can provide an analgesic basis in the peri-operative period. Under these circumstances, one can choose from drugs of different pharmacological classes, which all provide an analgesic effect.

Traditionally, to achieve an analgesic effect from the premedication phase onward, opioids are frequently used in dogs, although alpha2-

agonists such as xylazine, romifidine and medetomidine (availability depending on national licensing) can be viewed as good alternatives. Both classes of drugs can provide, depending on intrinsic potency and the dose administered, a solid analgesic basis upon which a surgical anaesthesia can be achieved with drugs such as hypnotics, dissociatives or volatiles. Although for most interventions, the duration of effects of the analgesic drugs will be adequately long (duration of analgesia: medetomidine ± 1 hour, methadone ± 1 hour, fentanyl ± 0.5 hour), one needs to consider redosing when the intervention exceeds the duration of action of the drug(s) employed.

In acute pain states in canines, as can be seen following trauma, opioid agonist drugs such as morphine, methadone or fentanyl can be used to effectively combat the most severe elements of pain. Due to the fact that in many of these cases, stress may be an important negative influence, these opioid agonists can be effectively combined with one of the major or minor tranquillisers. Adequate intravenous dosing of a 'neurolept-analgesic' combination such as morphine (or methadone) with acepromazine, fentanyl with droperidol, or methadone with diazepam (or midazolam) will effectively combat the pain while at the same time inducing a state of sedation which may well benefit the patient and consulting veterinarian as well.

Obviously, since most sedative agents will have dose-dependent cardiovascular side effects, the specific characteristics of these side effects will have to be considered when determining the indication for sedative administration, as well as the sedative drug of choice.

When continued intensive analgesic therapy is warranted, repeated administration or continuous low-dose i.v. administration of the same drugs or, alternatively, fentanyl patches may be considered.

Depending on the size of the patient and based upon a dose guideline of 2 - 4 μg/kg/h, one can choose from patches releasing 25 to 100 μg/h. Research has shown that fentanyl patches in dogs provide good analgesia [1] and ensure an adequate and fairly constant plasma level from 24 to 72 hours after application [2].

More recently, NSAIDs have been introduced for peri-operative pain relief. This group of pharmacological agents was traditionally used for treating chronic pain in dogs, especially that of an orthopaedic nature. The primary reason limiting the use of these drugs in the pre- and per-operative phase was related to their mechanism of action. Next to reduction of pain, all NSAIDs will inhibit prostaglandins involved in regulating renal perfusion (see also Chapter 6). As a consequence, the use of these drugs in circumstances such as anaesthesia, involving hypotension and reduced circulation, increases the risk of renal damage. It is therefore generally advised to limit the use of 6s to the post-operative period, and refrain from usage in patients with pre-existing cardiovascular, renal or gastrointestinal pathology. For the recently released carprofen, these limitations are of less importance, although potential side effects can never be ruled out altogether. Extensive field trials performed with carprofen support this proposed (gastro-intestinal and) renal safety, even when used pre-operatively [3].

Especially under those surgical circumstances where an activation of an inflammatory process can be foreseen, like interventions in arthritic joints or under septic conditions, the pre-operative use of a NSAID could potentially help reduce the further activation of the inflammatory process and, as a consequence, of the entire pain system. Such a pre-operative administration could benefit any surgical patient, both with regard to pain in the post-operative period and to the overall improvement post-surgically [4, 5]. By limiting peripheral and central sensitisation, both during and after surgery, achieving maximal pain relief becomes more realistic. It remains without doubt that further demands for general anaesthesia (including the potential use of opioids or alpha2-adrenergic drugs) will be needed during the intervention itself.

To obtain adequate pain relief post-operatively by systemic drug administration, one can choose between the administration of an opioid (such as buprenorphine) and a NSAID. Especially in those cases where the pain originates from surgery in non-inflamed tissue (such as elective abdominal surgery), the instalment of an opioid analgesic during the first 24-36 hours has been suggested to be most effective. In the time period following that, best results are most often obtained with the use of NSAIDs, which is explained on the basis of the interaction of the NSAID with the (sterile) inflammatory process that will follow any surgical trauma.

In those cases where the post-surgical pain is (expected to be) very intense, a polymodal therapy combining opioid and NSAID treatment, and in specific cases supported by local analgesic therapy, may be most beneficial to the patient.

For routine post-operative analgesic therapy following major surgical interventions (laparotomy, mammary gland resection) an initial opioid (buprenorphine) treatment for 24 hours, should be (combined and) followed up with medication for 2-4 days with one of the newer NSAIDs such as carprofen, vedaprofen, meloxicam or ketoprofen.

Chronic pain control

Taking into account the role that inflammation plays in the initiation and continued activation of pain processes, it becomes obvious that in chronic pain control the reduction of the inflammation is most prominent. Consequently, opioids can be expected to be less effective than NSAIDs, since the mechanism of action of the latter is based on an anti-inflammatory effect.

Generally speaking, it can be stated that the different NSAIDs that have been released onto the veterinary market in the recent years all exhibit a greater safety profile than the older alternatives from the same class of drugs. Within the group of relatively new non-steroidal anti-inflammatory agents, ketoprofen, meloxicam, vedaprofen and carprofen are all registered for multiple-day usage in dogs in one or more countries.

Specific drug classes employed for canine analgesic therapy

For the management of pain in canine patients, therapeutic agents come from one of the following three classes of drugs:

1   Centrally acting opioid agents, such as the different agonists (morphine, oxymorphone, methadone, fentanyl, pethidine), and the opioid partial agonist (buprenorphine), the agonist/antagonist (butorphanol, pentazocine, nalbuphine)

II *Substances that block the transport of impulses from nociceptors, either locally or centrally, such as local analgesics and the alpha-adrenergic agents like xylazine, romifidine and medetomidine.*

III *Agents that inhibit the production of the chemical inflammatory mediators activating (peripheral or central) pain pathways.*

Opioid analgesics (Table 1)

As a rule, opioids are considered to be the more potent analgesics. Due to the great variability in analgesic potency in (non-opioid) analgesics, the difference in analgesic potency between opioids and non-opioids has been lessened by the introduction of the new and more potent NSAIDs.

Opioids are primarily used for treatment of acute pain as well as peri-operatively for effectively controlling surgery-related pain. Its use does potentially cause some side effects that may potentially limit

Table 1
Selected dosages for opioids in dogs

Opioid	Dose in mg/kg	Duration	Route
Morphine	0.5-2	2-4 h	s.c.,i.m.
Pethidine	2-6	1-2 h	s.c.,i.m.
Oxymorphone	0.01-0.2	3-5 h	s.c.,i.m.,i.v.
Fentanyl	0.04-0.08	1-2 h	s.c.,i.m.,i.v.
Methadone	0.5-1.0	2-4 h	s.c.,i.m.
Buprenorphine	0.006-0.015	6-10 h	s.c.,i.m.
Butorphanol	0.2-0.4	2-5 h	s.c.,i.m.,i.v.
Nalbuphine	0.5-2.0	3-8 h	s.c.,i.m.,i.v.
Pentazocine	2.0-3.0	3-5 h	i.m.

opioid use under specific conditions. Side effects related to opioid usage include respiratory depression, increased intracranial pressure, and cardiovascular and behavioural effects. When used at the clinical dose levels in animals, the extent of these side effects does not prohibit the effective use of opioids as analgesic agents.

For the class of opioid analgesics, a differentiation can be made on the basis of either the specific opioid receptor (μ, κ and δ) affinity, or the agonist-antagonist character of the opioids, separating the agonist opioids (like morphine, oxymorphone, methadone, fentanyl and pethidine), from the partial agonist (buprenorphine) and mixed agonist/antagonist opioids (like nalbuphine, pentazocine and butorphanol).

Under most circumstances, the use of agonist agents is limited to the pre- and per-anaesthetic period, and it is combined with a tranquilliser such as acepromazine, droperidol or diazepam/ midazolam, to produce adequate premedication or even full neurolept-analgesic anaesthesia.

Generally speaking, the longer acting agonist opioids like morphine, methadone and pethidine are much less potent analgesics than fentanyl, and are more likely to produce respiratory and/or cardiovascular side effects. The more potent analgesic fentanyl, on the other hand, has a limited duration of action (< 30 min) and as a consequence for prolonged procedures this agent must be repeatedly (or continuously) administered.

For extended pain relief (> 3-4 h), whether it is following general anaesthesia or not, the partial agonist or the mixed agonist/antagonist opioids are commonly used in a wide variety of species including the dog [6, 7]. Although there is the possibility of the development of tolerance following opioid administration, this usually occurs only after several days of treatment, and may then result in an inadequate pain relief.

The partial agonist and mixed agonist/antagonist opioid agents (like buprenorphine, nalbuphine, pentazocine and butorphanol) either demonstrate their dual influence on a single type of receptor (i.e. buprenorphine on the μ-receptor [subtypes?]), or have an agonistic effect on one, and an antagonistic effect on another type of receptor (i.e. nalbuphine shows μ-receptor antagonism and κ-receptor agonism). Their dual character of action makes these agents especially useful in pain control following anaesthesia, since their effect combines antagonism of the sedative and respiratory depressant effect, while their agonistic action ensures an analgesic effect. All these mixed agonist/antagonist opioid drugs are (relatively) long acting, and a bell-shaped dose response curve has been described for most of them. This latter quality does not interfere with the possibility of obtaining adequate analgesia under clinical circumstances (see also Chapter 6).

Buprenorphine couples a slow onset (15-30 min) with a duration of action of 8-10 h and a good analgesic effect with little sedative, cardiovascular or respiratory side-effects [8]. This combination of effects makes it excellently suitable for achieving post-anaesthetic analgesia in different species. Similar results are obtained with pentazocine, although this agent has a weaker potency and a shorter duration of action (approximately 4 h) than buprenorphine.

Butorphanol has an intermediate analgesic potency, with duration of action similar to that of pentazocine. Both butorphanol and buprenorphine have been documented to occasionally induce sedation in dogs while much less [8], if any, behavioural changes are seen with the use of nalbuphine [9].

Next to the systemic administration of opioid drugs, local application can greatly improve the patient's condition by reducing the intensity of the pain and preventing, or at the very least limiting, the onset of hypersensitisation of the pain system.

Examples of such local opioid application are the epidural administration of opioids such as morphine [10]at a dose of 0.1 mg/kg and oxymorphone at 0.15 mg/kg [11], possibly combined with an α2-agonist. Also, a single post-surgery intra-articular administration of morphine has been shown to have pain-reducing effect for the first 24 h following cruciate ligament repair in dogs [12].

Local anaesthetics

Although a wide variety of applications of local anaesthetics in relieving pain in animals can be accrued, the character of many our canine patients prevents the large-scale use of local anaesthetics as a single anaesthetic agent. The most commonly used local anaesthetics are lidocaine (lignocaine) and bupivacaine, although others are available and their use is occasionally described in the veterinary literature. Lidocaine, used in a concentration of 1-2%, pairs a fast onset of action (5-10 min) with a relative short duration of effect (45-60 min). Its effect can be prolonged by the addition of adrenaline (1:100,000 or 1:200,000), which reduces the absorption of the local anaesthetic from the site of injection and thereby prolongs its effect. Bupivacaine 0.75% combines a slow onset of action (10-20 min) with an effect that may last up to 3 h.

Instead of the use of local anaesthetics as sole or primary anaesthetic, a more practical approach is the application of local analgesics in a combination of sedation/light anaesthesia with the local application of a local analgesic to maximise the alleviation of pain. This can be achieved with a single-dose administration of a short- or long-acting, local analgesic (nerve block, infiltration analgesia), or by repeated or continuous administration with an epidural catheter.

An effective local anaesthetic effect can allow a significant reduction of necessary anaesthetic depth or an improved quality of analgesia per-operatively and during recovery. This can be achieved with an epidural administration of long-acting drugs like bupivacaine [13] or intra-articular administered bupivacaine [12]. Other examples include the brachial plexus block prior to limb amputation which decreases the noxious impulse barrage to the spinal cord, thereby preventing full blown sensitisation from occurring, or the installation of a long acting local anaesthetic such as bupivacaine (1.5 mg/kg) interpleurally, to combat the pain following thoracotomy [14].

Alpha-adrenergic agents

The agents from the class of α2-adrenergic drugs, like xylazine, romifidine and medetomidine, can be categorised as being sedative/ analgesic, and consequently clearly induce a state of sedation together with the analgesia [15].

On account of the sedative/analgesic effect, the use of α2-adrenergic drugs is primarily limited to general anaesthesia in various animal species where these agents, and especially the potent medetomidine, greatly reduce the required dose of any concurrently administered anaesthetic drug [16].

Next to the sedation and analgesia, drugs from this class produce significant cardiovascular side-effects which include initial hypertension, followed by normo-/hypotension, increased peripheral resistance, a decreased heart rate and cardiac output. Like opioids and local analgesics, alpha2-drugs, and especially medetomidine, have been successfully administered epidurally [11] at a dose of 10–15 µg/kg.

It has been shown that medetomidine, administered epidurally, can provide a long-lasting analgesia when administered on its own, but also that it can significantly prolong (and potentially intensify) the analgesia induced by epidurally administered morphine in dogs.

Non-steroidal anti-inflammatory drugs (Table 2)

With a weak analgetic potency ascribed to the earlier NSAIDs, the more recently developed NSAIDs have sufficient analgesic potency to effectively combat peri-operative pain and might thereby be attractive alternatives for opioids in the post-operative phase, whenever the latter are contra-indicated. Also, the anti-inflammatory effects of NSAIDs provide for specific indications within the polymodal 'pain-control' protocol in the post-surgery period, since inflammation usually develops within several hours after the intervention (see Chapter 5). Where NSAIDs were traditionally seen as peripherally acting analgesics, recent evidence clearly suggests these drugs to have a central effect at the level of the spinal cord as well [17, 18].

Table 2

Selected dosages for NSAIDs in dogs

NSAIDs	Dose in mg/kg	Duration	Route
Acetylsalicylic Acid	10-20	12 h	Orally
Phenylbutazone	10-15	12 h	i.v.
Phenylbutazone	10-20	24 h	Orally
Flunixine	0.5-1.0	24 h	i.m.,i.v.
Tolfenamic acid	4	48 h	s.c., i.m.
Tolfenamic acid	3-5	24 h	Orally
Ibuprofen	10	24 h	Orally
Ketoprofen	2 first day 1 following days	24 h	s.c., i.m., i.v.
Ketoprofen	1	24 h	Orally
Dipyrone (Metamizol)	25	12 h	s.c., i.m., i.v.
Meloxicam	0.2	24 h	Orally
Vedaprofen	0.5	24 h	Orally
Carprofen	2	12 h	Orally
Carprofen	2-4	Once pre-operatively	s.c., i.v.
Ketorolac	0.5	12 h	i.m., i.v.

In addition to their analgesic, anti-inflammatory and anti-pyretic effects, NSAIDs may also produce unwanted side effects. Following repeated administration, the most prominent side effect is the gastro-intestinal irritation that may subsequently lead to gastroduodenal ulceration. A large part of these side effects are ascribed to the differential effects NSAIDs exert on cyclo-oxygenase (COX) type I and cyclo-oxygenase (COX) type II. The negative side effects are then primarily dependent on the reduction of the formation of the constituent COX I, although new insights now provide evidence that this presents a clear oversimplification, and further research is needed to fully elucidate this.

Despite the above, it is clear that under circumstances of reduced circulation (due to underlying pathology or on account of general anaesthesia), renal perfusion may be diminished due to an absent or decreased regulatory effect of circulating prostaglandins. It is this characteristic that presents the major contraindication for the pre-operative use of NSAIDs in dogs. The major exception to this rule is carprofen, which combines good efficacy with little or no side effects. As a consequence, this drug is at present the only NSAID registered for pre-operative administration in canine patients in several countries. Although it has been suggested that the same holds true for meloxicam, formal proof of this has yet to be shown and no official registration for its pre-operative use has yet been realised.

References

1   Robinson TM, Kruse-Elliot KT, Markel MD, Pluhar GE, Massa K, Bjorling DE. A comparison of transdermal fentanyl versus epidural morphine for analgesia in dogs undergoing major orthopedic surgery. J Am Anim Hosp Assoc 1999;35:95-100.
2   Kyles AE, Papich M, Hardie EM. Disposition of transdermally administered fentanyl in dogs. Am J Vet Res 1996;57:715-9.
3   Lascelles BD, Butterworth SJ, Waterman-Pearson AE. Postoperative analgesic and sedative effects of carprofen and pethidine in dogs. Vet Rec 1994;134:187-91.
4   Lascelles BD, Cripps PJ, Jones A, Waterman-Pearson AE. Efficacy and kinetics of carprofen, administered preoperatively or postoperatively, for the prevention of pain in dogs undergoing ovariohysterctomy. Vet Surg 1998;27:568-82.
5   Grisneaux E, Pibarot P, Dupuis J, Blais D. Comparison of ketoprofen and carprofen administered prior to orthopedic surgery for control of postoperative pain in dogs. J Am Vet Med Assoc 1999; 215:1105-10.
6   Hellyer PW. Management of acute and surgical pain. Semin Vet Med Surg (Small Anim) 1997;12:106-14.
7   Taylor PM. Newer analgesics. Nonsteroid anti-inflammatory drugs, opioids, and combinations. Vet Clin North Am Small Anim Pract 1999;29:719-35.

8   Cowan A, Doxey JC, Harry EJ. The animal pharmacology of buprenorphine, an oripavine analgesic agent. Brit J Pharmacol 1977; 60:547-54.

9   Schmidt WK, Tam SW, Shotzberger GS, Smith DH, Clark R, Vernier VG. Nalbuphine. Drug Alcohol Depend 1985;14:339-62.

10 Keegan RD, Greene SA, Weil AB. Cardiovascular effects of epidurally administered morphine and a xylazine-morphine combination in isoflurane-anesthetized dogs. Am J Vet Res 1995;56:496-500.

11 Vesal N, Cribb PH, Frketic M. Postoperative analgesic and cardiopulmonary effects in dogs of oxymorphone administered epidurally and intramuscularly, and medetomidine administered epidurally: a comparative clinical study. Vet Surg 1996;25:361-9.

12 Sammarco JL, Conzemius MG, Perkowski SZ, Weinstein MJ, Grehor TP, Smith GK. Postoperative analgesia for stifle surgery: a comparison of intra-articular bupivacaine, morphine and saline. Vet Surg 1996;25:59-69.

13 Heath RB, Broadstone RV, Wright M, Grandy JL. Using bupivacaine hydrochloride for lumbosacral epidural analgesia. Compendium Sm Anim 1989;11:50-5.

14 Flecknell PA, Kirk AJ, Liles JH, Hayes PH, Dark JH. Postoperative analgesia following thoracotomy in the dog: an evaluation of the effects of bupivacaine intercostal nerve block and nalbuphine on respiratory function. Lab Anim 1991;25:319-24.

15 Vaha-Vahe T. Clinical evaluation of medetomidine, a novel sedative and analgesic drug for dogs and cats. Acta Vet Scand 1989;30:267-73.

16 Vickery RG, Sheridan BC, Segal IS, Maze M. Anesthetic and hemodynamic effects of the stereoisomers of medetomidine, an alpha-2 adrenergic agonist, in halothane-anesthetized dogs. Anesth Analg 1988;67:611-5.

17 Cashman JN. The mechanisms of action of NSAIDs in analgesia. Drugs 1996;52:13-23.

18 Herrero JF, Parrado A, Cervero F. Central and peripheral actions of the NSAID ketoprofen on spinal cord nociceptive reflexes. Neuropharmacol 1997;36:1425-31.

8

MANAGEMENT OF PAIN IN CATS

Karol A. Mathews, Ontario Veterinary College,
University of Guelph, Guelph, Canada

Introduction

During the last decade, great strides have been made in the assessment and treatment of pain, or its prevention, in both human and veterinary medicine. It is known that animals feel, and anticipate, pain by similar mechanisms as humans do [1] (Chapters 2 & 5). The presence of pain in animals also has both physiological [2,3] and emotional effects (personal observations), similar to those in people. Continual painful experience in any animal is detrimental to the overall healing process as well as to the general well-being. This is especially so in cats, where problems such as hepatic lipidosis may occur due to inappetance and inadequate caloric intake. Based on recent surveys of animal health technicians in Canada [4] and veterinarians in Canada [5], Britain [6] and Australasia [7], caregivers appear to administer analgesics less frequently to cats than to dogs.

The potential toxicity or adverse reactions associated with these drugs is a major concern of most veterinarians. However, with the current knowledge of the pharmacology and defined, rather than hypothesised, adverse effects of some analgesics in cats [8] (Chapter 6) this should no longer be a reason for non-analgesic use in cats. Another reason for non-analgesic use in cats is that pain is difficult to recognise, especially in chronic painful situations, but even this can be identified with experience (Chapter 4). However, where acute pain is present, such as post-surgical or traumatic pain, certain behavioural characteristics are present and readily apparent [9] (Chapter 4). One should become familiar with the subtle signs of pain signalling the early onset of mild to moderate pain, where analgesic therapy will prevent the development of worse pain which is more difficult to control [9]. Based on physiological and anatomical similarities of pain perception and processing, an anthropomorphic approach to management of pain may be employed when behavioural characteristics cannot be readily recognised.

The key points in treatment of pain in cats are:
- *to think in terms of the similarities of pain perception in both humans and cats and treat with an analgesic appropriate for the level of pain likely to be present. Age also contributes to behavioural patterns associated with pain, whereby younger animals tend to be more vocal.*
- *to be familiar with the various drug treatment modalities proven to be safe and effective in this species, both in health and disease.*
- *to recognise (both subtle and obvious) signs and behaviour associated with pain; keeping in mind that cats tend to withdraw and remain quiet through a wide range of painful experiences.*

In considering these, the veterinarian will gain experience in treating pain in cats. Administration of analgesics may also be diagnostic in those situations where pain behaviour is difficult to recognise.

There are many analgesics available, which may or may not be licensed in various countries, which are safe and effective in cats. Off-label use of analgesics is common practice; therefore, it is suggested to search for guidelines in analgesic use rather than be limited to specific 'licensed' drugs in the individual countries.

Several groups of analgesics may be administered to cats.
1 *Opioids, comprising pure agonists (oxymorphone, hydromorphone, morphine, fentanyl, meperidine or pethidine, and codeine are the most common), partial agonists (buprenorphine) or agonist-antagonists (butorphanol)* [6, 10];
2 *non-steroidal anti-inflammatory drugs (NSAIDs) (carprofen, ketoprofen, meloxicam, tolfenamic acid, flunixin meglumine, ketorolac tromethamine)* [6,9];
3 *local anaesthetics (lidocaine, bupivicaine, mepivicaine)* [11];
4 *alpha2-agonists (xylazine, medetomidine - medetomidine antagonist atipamezole), effective for pre-emptive analgesic use and selected cases of pain management* [6, 12];
5 *ketamine, while not commonly used as an analgesic, may be used for*

peracute pain management [6] or, when short-term (i.e. head trauma requiring re-assessment) analgesia is required where opioids are not available or adequate and

6 *the chondroprotective drugs which may be beneficial for the treatment of osteoarthritis [13-15].*

With respect to dosing, there is no ceiling effect with the pure opioids which permits titration of dose to (analgesic) effect. The opioid partial agonists or agonist-antagonists do have a ceiling effect where giving more may actually reduce the analgesic effect. With NSAIDs, administration must not exceed the recommended dose due to the potential adverse effects. Also, NSAIDs should be titrated down to effect to obtain the lowest dose possible to alleviate pain while reducing the potential of adverse effects when used long term.

In general, very young or geriatric patients [16] or those with liver or renal disease should receive the lower to average dosage of an opioid analgesic initially, with additional doses slowly titrated intravenously (i.v.) to the desired effect. A specific, fixed dose cannot be recommended, as the level of pain may vary and many of these animals may ultimately require the same dose as any other animal. It is important to realise the potential degree of pain the cat may be experiencing, as the selection of the appropriate analgesic depends on this. Selecting an opioid partial agonist or agonist-antagonist to treat severe pain can be detrimental. Not only does this not confer sufficient analgesia, it can potentially prevent the efficacy of the pure opioid subsequently administered in an attempt to control severe pain.

Frequently it is impossible to administer oral analgesics to cats and often pills or capsules are formulated in large doses making accurate administration difficult. Exceptions are meloxicam formulated in a palatable syrup and glucosamine/chondroitin sulphate that can be sprinkled on the food. Codeine and morphine can be formulated in a malt syrup or fish paste, both palatable to cats.

Acute pain management

The management of acute pain frequently requires 'acute' treatment in that the analgesic administered should have an (almost) immediate effect (Table 1). For peracute management of pain, morphine, oxymorphone, hydromorphone, fentanyl, ketamine combined with midazolam or diazepam (both at 0.1–0.3 mg/kg), can be titrated i.v. to effect. It is advisable to leave the i.v. catheter in place whilst the cat is recovering to manage potential acute pain. The preferred routes of administration of morphine are intramuscularly (i.m.) or subcutaneously (s.c.); however, it can be administered i.v. if given very slowly [10] or rectally. For moderate pain (Table 1), lower doses of the pure opioids or butorphanol are adequate. Meperidine may be acceptable for use initially with a prolonged analgesic regimen after patient assessment. Where i.v. access cannot be obtained in the injured or painful cat, ketamine 2-10 mg/kg can be sprayed onto the oral mucous membranes. When possible, place an indwelling i.v. catheter and administer midazolam or diazepam and connect to a continuous delivery system of a balanced electrolyte solution to facilitate drug administration at a distance from the cat. To reduce the pain and facilitate i.v. catheter placement, apply a topical anesthetic

Table 1
Suggested analgesics for the initial management of acute pain in cats

Moderate to severe pain

Drug	Dose	Duration of action
Morphine	0.1-0.2+ mg/g i.m.,s.c.	2-6 h
Oxymorphone	0.02-0.1+ mg/kg i.v., i.m., s.c.	2-6 h
Hydromorphone	0.1-0.3+ mg/kg i.v., i.m., s.c.	2-6 h
Fentanyl	0.001–0.004+ mg/kg	0.3 h
Ketamine	1-4 mg/kg i.v.	
	5-10 mg/kg p.o.	prn (~0.5 h)

Mild to moderate pain

Butorphanol	0.1–0.4 i.v.	
	0.4-0.8 mg/kg i.m., s.c.	2-3 h
Meperidine (pethidine)	5-10 mg/kg i.m., s.c.	20 – 30 min

Table 2

Suggested analgesia for post-operative or dental pain

Moderate to severe pain

Drug	Dose	Duration of action
Morphine	0.1-0.2+ mg/kg i.v.	1-4 h
	0.1-0.5 i.m., s.c.	2-6 h
Oxymorphone	0.02-0.05+ mg/kg i.v.	2–4 h or
	0.05–0.2 i.m., s.c.	2–6 h
Hydromorphone	0.1-0.3 mg/kg i.v., i.m., s.c.	2-6 h
Fentanyl	0.004–0.01+ mg/kg i.v. bolus	0.3 h
	0.001–0.004+ mg/kg/h	CRI
Fentanyl patch	2 µg (may require suppl. analgesia)	
Ketoprofen	2 mg/kg s.c.	Initially, then
	1.0 mg/kg	every 24 h up to 4 days
Meloxicam	0.3 mg/kg s.c.	Initially, then
	0.1 mg/kg	every 24 h up to 4 days
Carprofen	4.0 mg/kg s.c.	Once
Flunixin meglumine	1.0 mg/kg s.c.	Once
Ketorolac trimethamine	0.25 mg/kg i.m.	Repeat once 8-12 h

Mild to moderate pain

Drug	Dose	Duration of action
Opioids above	Low dosages	
NSAIDs above	Low dosages	Titrate down
Butorphanol	0.4-0.8 mg/kg	2-3 h
Meperidine(pethidine)*	5-10 mg/kg i.m., s.c. administered at time of NSAID injection.	20–30 min
Morphine syrup	0.5 mg/kg p.o. - titrate to effect	Every 4-6 h
Codeine	0.5-2mg/kg p.o. - titrate to effect	Every 6-12 h
Bupivicaine 0.5%	1 mg/kg (0.2 ml/kg lean weight) + 0.02mEq/kg sodium bicarbonate diluted to 12 ml with saline for intra-pleural and peritoneal use	2-6 h

Sedatives to be combined with opioids

Drug	Dose	Duration of action
Midazolam	0.1–0.5 mg/kg i.v., i.m.	Up to 6 h
Diazepam	0.1–0.5 mg/kg i.v.	Up to 6 h
Acepromazine	0.01-0.03 mg/kg i.v.	1-2 h
	0.02–0.1 mg/kg i.m., s.c.	2-6 h

* Not suitable as an analgesic alone due to short duration of action cream, such as lignocaine-prilocaine (EMLA cream, Astra), over the previously shaved and cleansed venipuncture site, approximately 15-20 min prior to catheterisation.

In addition to analgesics, sedatives may be useful in settling the anxious patient (Table 2). Sedatives have no intrinsic analgesic properties; in fact pain perception may be heightened if used alone.

With respect to ongoing acute, painful medical conditions, such as pancreatitis, meningitis, accidental hypothermia (painful on re-warming for ($\geq$72 hours) or surgical pain, analgesics should be administered prior to the onset of moderate to severe pain (Table 2). It is well understood that pre-emptive analgesia reduces nociceptive facilitation and central nervous system sensitisation that ultimately

Table 3

Pre-emptive use of analgesics in cats

Drug	Dose	Duration of action
Those in Table 1		
Lidocaine 1%	1.5-2 mg/kg (0.2 ml/kg) divided for neural blockade	0.3 h
Bupivicaine 0.25%	1 mg/kg (0.4 ml/kg) divided for neural blockade	2-6 h
Medetomidine	0.001-0.01 mg/kg i.v., i.m., s.c.	0.5–2 h
Xylazine	0.1–1 mg/kg i.v., i.m., s.c.	0.5–2 h
Epidural Solutions	0.2 ml/kg	4-8 h
2% Lidocaine	alone or with opioid*	
2% Mepivacaine	alone or with opioid*	
0.5% Bupivacaine	alone or with opioid*	
Morphine	0.1mg/kg**	
Oxymorphone	0.05 mg/kg**	
Hydromorphone	0.03 mg/kg**	

* Obtain opioid dose first, then add the local anaesthetic to a total of 0.2 ml/kg

** If opioid without local anaesthetic is required, dilute with sterile saline to a total volume of 0.2 ml/kg.

reduces the experience of pain. Various techniques and analgesic regimens may be used in this regard [11, 16](Table 3).

The dosages and duration of action of most analgesics are average recommendations and may not be adequate for severe to excruciating pain. For example, where morphine is noted to last 4-6 hours in cats, this may not be so in severe pain when using 0.2 mg/kg, and a higher dose or more frequent administration may be necessary. Continuous monitoring is required and recognition of subtle signs of pain should guide the repeat dosing. For continuous delivery of analgesia, a constant rate infusion (CRI) can be established by taking the previous dose and duration of action, and delivering this amount over a similar time period. This can be titrated up or down depending on the patient's response. The major drawback to the CRI is delivering the opioid i.v. to patients who are not continually supervised. Opioids may cause heavy sedation when overdosed, requiring temporary cessation with reinstitution at a lower dose. Respiratory depression as a serious side effect of the opioids is over-emphasized (I have never noted this when animals are painful) and primarily extrapolated from the human setting. Opioids used in combination with sedatives as a form of chemical restraint in non-painful geriatric animals or with general anaesthesia can produce respiratory depression. Hypotension may result due to changes in heart rate or effects of the other drugs used. Morphine given i.v. as a bolus will cause hypotension and possibly excitement and vomiting. However, given as a slow push over five minutes in the painful patient these side effects may be avoided [10].

Pain frequently results in tachypnea; as opioids reduce the perception of pain, the respiratory rate is also lowered to within the normal range. Panting may occur with certain opioids, if the dose was excessive for the pain experienced. This is due to effects on the thermo-regulatory centre. Where head injury is causing pain, fentanyl is the analgesic of choice. Fentanyl's short duration of action allows neurological evaluation when the CRI is temporarily stopped or reduced. In these painful patients, ketamine 1-2 mg/kg i.v. and 0.05–0.1 mg/kg diazepam or midazolam i.v. as required may also be beneficial.

A transdermal fentanyl patch is an excellent delivery system for continuous administration of an analgesic in cats. Most cats require the 25 µg/h patch. The patch should not be cut and when a lower dose is required, only part of the seal is removed. The rate of delivery of fentanyl is only 30% of the theoretical level; therefore, overdose is unlikely to occur in the average-sized cat. The 25 µg/h patch requires 6-12 hours to reach therapeutic levels, which remain in steady state for approximately 5 days in most cats [17]. There is individual variation where adjunct analgesia is required for longer than 12 hours and again required before the fifth day. Morphine, oxymorphone, hydro-morphone or a low dose CRI of fentanyl are the supplemental analgesics of choice. Placement of the patch is usually on the dorsum of the lower part of the neck or between the scapulae on the intact, shaven skin. Adverse effects are similar to other opioids. The patch can be removed when adverse effects are noted and the reversal is fairly rapid (2–3 h). Naloxone titrated to effect (dilute 0.1 ml of 0.4 mg/ml naloxone in 9 ml saline and deliver at 1 ml increments up to 0.04 mg/CAT), may be given for more rapid removal if needed. Special care should be given when using these patches with regard to placement, misuse by other members of the household and disposal of the patch at the end of treatment.

Meperidine is adequate for mild to moderate pain. Due to its short duration of action, it is usually reserved for short term pain such as in cats with urethral obstruction during retropulsion [6]. It may also be used initially with concurrent administration of a NSAID, which usually takes 45–60 min to become effective. In my experience, the newer NSAIDs are excellent analgesics, frequently managing severe pain where the opioids have failed [10]. Meloxicam, carprofen, ketoprofen, tolfenamic acid, flunixin meglumine and ketorolac trimethamine are available in parenteral formulations. Once the acute pain patient is controlled with an opioid and assessed as having a normal cardiovascular, renal, hepatic and GI status, a NSAID may be administered [10]. Should pain control for more than one day be necessary, ketoprofen or meloxicam may be administered parenterally or orally. Where surgery is contemplated, the use of NSAIDs should be restricted to post-operative use until further studies prove the safety of pre-operative use in cats. The NSAIDs are excellent analgesics for both orthopaedic and soft tissue pain. Strict adherence to the maximum dosing regimen is necessary to avoid renal failure or gastrointestinal ulceration.

Preemptive analgesia, using multimodal analgesic regimens, can be designed to reduce surgical nociceptive input and subsequent post-operative pain [18](Table 3). The use of opioids as a pre-anaesthetic — medetomidine in the healthy patient, or ketamine combined with a benzodiazepine in the geriatric or unstable patient — are excellent for their antinociceptive actions. Should NSAIDs prove to be safe in cats when used preemptively, these too may be of benefit in this regard. Neural blockade using local anaesthetics, such as 0.25% bupivicaine at a maximum of 0.4 ml/kg divided to block all nerves involved, can be used to reduce post-operative pain [11]. Intercostal nerve block during thoracotomy is performed by infiltration of 0.25% bupivicaine on the posterior aspect of the rib close to the spinal column while avoiding the intercostal artery and spanning at least 2 intercostal spaces each side of the incision. During forelimb amputation, desensitisation of the brachial plexus may be carried out intraoperatively by infiltration of 0.25% bupivicaine 15 min prior to transection. Percutaneous desensitisation, after induction of anesthesia has been described [11]. Similar techniques should be applied to the femoral and sciatic nerves prior to hind limb amputation and ulnar nerve branches and the median nerve can be blocked percutaneously prior to onychectomy. Local anaesthetic, such as 1% lidocaine, should be used in high-risk patients prior to any emergency procedure (i.e. chest drain placement, venous cut down), which also reduces the pain perception when the animal's condition improves. Using a chest drain for intrapleural instillation, or a catheter for intraperitoneal instillation of 0.2 ml/kg of 0.5% bupivacaine with 0.02 mEq/kg of sodium bicarbonate diluted to 12 ml with 0.9% saline, is a useful adjunct to opioid analgesics for incisional pain – after thoracotomy – or pain associated with pancreatitis. Sodium bicarbonate reduces the pain from the local anaesthetic solution by increasing the pH. After administration, the animal should be placed with the injured side down for 5 min to enhance the local anaesthetic effect. Without the sodium bicarbonate, local anaesthetic within the pleural space or abdomen, is very painful.

Epidural analgesia is frequently used to prevent, reduce or treat pain in dogs. Its use in cats is encouraged to provide intraoperative and postoperative analgesia for procedures performed caudal to T 13 innervation (Table 3). Local anaesthesia is beneficial for immediate (5–15 min) sensation and motor blockade caudal to the lower thoracic segments (approaching the anterior abdomen). Morphine produces an effect (by 30–60 min) as far forward as the front limbs, and is unlikely to produce any respiratory effects. Oxymorphone is highly bound at the area of placement and therefore limits the analgesic effects to the posterior part of the body (onset by 30 min). Systemic effects (5–15 min) are often observed in the anaesthetised patient. Hydromorphone's pharmacokinetic behaviour is between morphine and oxymorphone and is used for preemptive analgesia in small animals (personal communication - D. Dyson, Ontario Veterinary College).

Occasionally, epidural analgesia may be chosen for the awake animal for long duration analgesia, reducing or potentially eliminating the requirement for systemic analgesics. Potential adverse effects associated with epidural analgesics are occasional vomiting with morphine, late onset respiratory depression (rarely) and urinary retention. Contraindications for this procedure are sepsis, coagulation disorders (NSAID therapy!) or skin infection near the site for injection. For detailed information on this technique the reader is referred to the relevant veterinary literature.

For moderate pain, the lower doses of the pure opioid given i.v., i.m. or s.c. are usually adequate, with additional dosing if needed. For mild pain, the pure opioids are excessive and may cause excitement if doses in excess of minimal are used. It is advised to titrate the dose to effect and, if overdose occurs, reversal agents such as naloxone can be titrated in small increments (up to a dose of 0.04 mg/kg i.v.) to remove the unwanted effects. The duration of action of opioids is longer than naloxone; therefore, naloxone titration may have to be repeated. Analgesia may be preserved using this technique.

Butorphanol or buprenorphine are appropriate analgesics for mild to moderate acute pain such as the early stages of pancreatitis or following ovariohysterectomy [19]. The duration of effect is short (~ 2–4 hours) for butorphanol, requiring repeat administration. The onset of action of buprenorphine requires up to 45 minutes with a reported duration of action to be 12 hours; however, in practice, it is more predictably 6 hours and occasionally ineffective [6]. Codeine can be administered after various surgical procedures where NSAIDs are contraindicated. Otherwise, ketoprofen or meloxicam for 4 days may be administered for post-operative pain. The recommended analgesic regimen for tooth extraction in these patients is to use an opioid pre-anaesthetic and local anesthetic blockade of the appropriate nerves with bupivicaine 0.25% [11]. Where there are no contraindications, NSAIDs may be administered upon extubation, where haemorrhage is a concern, ketoprofen and Aspirin must be avoided. Codeine or morphine for more painful patients, both in syrup or paste formulations, may be administered orally for at least 12 to 24 hours or more, as soon as the cat is able to swallow.

Chronic pain management

Chronic pain may be difficult to recognise, as it is frequently insidious in onset. The owners may present their cat with a history of reduced appetite, weight loss, reluctance to move, not grooming, or it may have a noticeable limp. Inflammatory joint disease in the cat has

Table 4

Suggested treatment for chronic pain (>5 days) in cats

Drug	Dose	Duration of action
Fentanyl 'patch'	25 μg/h	as needed up to every 5 days
Meloxicam	0.3 mg/kg s.c., p.o.	Once
	0.1 mg/kg p.o.	daily for 4 days, then
	0.1 mg/CAT p.o.	alternate days
Codeine	0.5–2.0 mg/kg p.o.	Every 8-12 h
Morphine syrup	0.5 mg/kg p.o.	Every 4-6 h
Aspirin	10–20 mg/kg p.o.	Every 48 h
Corticosteroids	1-2 mg/kg	Every 24 h, reducing daily dose based on the underlying disease

many etiologies including infection, immune-mediated, degenerative and traumatic [13]. The cause must be identified as the treatment varies with the aetiology (Table 4).

Where immune-mediated disease is diagnosed, prednisone or prednisolone at 2 mg/kg q 12-24 h initially, is the treatment of choice. Medical management for osteoarthritis includes weight loss in obese cats, lowering the food and water bowl and bed to floor level to avoid further trauma to the joints, and pain management. Chondro-protective drugs and cartilage preparations have been reported to provide effective treatment in these cats [13-15]. Meloxicam 0.3 mg/kg once, followed by 0.1 mg/kg q 24 h for 4 days or ketoprofen 2 mg/kg once, followed by 0.5 to 1.0 mg/kg q 24 h for 4 days has shown to be effective in acute or chronic locomotor disorders in cats [6]. For more chronic use, meloxicam 0.1 mg/CAT/q 2 days is routinely used in veterinary practice in Britain with no reported adverse effects (personal communication – A.Henderson, Boehringer-Ingelheim, UK). However, as no prospective, controlled studies using meloxicam chronically have been conducted, it is recommended that intermittent assessment of renal and hepatic function be carried out. Meloxicam appears not to interfere with the synthesis of cartilage proteoglycans [20], which is a potential problem with other NSAIDs such as Aspirin. Aspirin has been recommended for chronic osteoarthritic pain in cats [13, 19]. As with all NSAIDs, gastro-intestinal side effects may occur. It is always advisable to reduce the dose to the lowest possible level that maintains analgesia. Pain associated with cancer can be treated chronically with morphine 0.5mg/kg q 4 - 6 initially with titration to effect (either lower or higher) based on the cat's behaviour (personal communication - J. Gaynor, Colorado State University) or fentanyl transdermal patch. Many medical problems such as cystitis, meningitis or otitis are painful and analgesics may be administered while treating the primary condition. A low dose of NSAIDs is recommended in these conditions, with gradual reduction and discontinuation as the primary problem resolves. However, the co-administration of NSAIDs with corticosteroids must be avoided. NSAIDs may be administered to cats in combination with opioids to avoid using the higher doses of each analgesic if used alone, as well as being more effective than each one alone for severe pain, i.e. cancer pain.

In conclusion, pain is present in many medical, surgical and traumatic conditions in cats as well as in dogs and humans. The demonstration of pain is not as obvious in cats and therefore pain should be assumed in any condition producing pain in other species. Response to analgesic administration can guide the veterinarian in the management of pain (or presumed pain). This practice will allow the practitioner to gain experience in recognizing and treating pain in cats.

References

1 Vierck CJ. Extrapolation from the pain research literature to problems of adequate veterinary care. J Am Vet Med Assoc 1976;168:510-4.
2 Smith JD, Allen SW, Quandt JE, Tackett RL. Indicators of postoperative pain in cats and correlation with clinical criteria. Am J Vet Res 1996;209:1674-8.
3 Benson GJ, Wheaton LG, Thurmon JC, Tranquilli WJ, Olson WA, Davis CA. Postoperative catecholamine response to onychectomy in isoflurane-anesthetized cats: Effect of analgesics. Vet Surg 1991;20(3):222-5.
4 Dohoo SE, Dohoo IR. Attitudes and concerns of Canadian animal health technologists toward postoperative pain management in dogs and cats. Can Vet J 1998;39:491-6.
5 Dohoo SE, Dohoo IR. Factors influencing the postoperative use of analgesics in dogs and cats by Canadian veterinarians. Can Vet J 1996;37:552-6.
6 Lascelles BDX, Waterman A. Analgesia in cats. In Practice 1997;19(4)203-13.
7 Watson ADJ, Nicholson A, Church DB, Pearson MRB. Use of anti-inflammatory and analgesic drugs in dogs and cats. Aust Vet J 1996;74:203-10.
8 Wilcke JR. Idiosyncracies of drug metabolism in cats: Effects on pharmacotherapeutics in feline practice. Vet Clin N Am Sm Anim Prac 1984;14(6):1345-54.
9 Mathews KA. Non-steroidal anti-inflammatory analgesics for acute pain management in dogs and cats. Vet Comp Traum Ortho 1997;10:122-9.
10 Hellyer PW, Gaynor JS. Acute post-surgical pain in dogs and cats. Comp Cont Educ Pract Vet 1998;20(2):140-53.

11 Skarda RT. Local and regional anesthetic and analgesic techniques: In: Thurmon JC. Tranquilli WJ, Benson GJ (Eds). 'Lumb and Jones' Veterinary Anesthesia, Williams and Wilkins, Baltimore, MD,1996:426-47.

12 Cullen LK. Medetomidine sedation in dogs and cats: A review of its pharmacology, antagonism and dose. Br Vet J 1996;152:519-35.

13 Hardie EM. Management of osteoarthtirits in cats. Vet Clin N Am Sm Anim Prac 1997;27(4):945-53.

14 Kyles AE, Ruslander D. Chronic pain: Osteoarthritis and cancer. Sem Vet Med Surg Sm Anim 1997;12(2):122-32.

15 Kendall RK. Therapeutic nutrition for the cat, dog and horse. In: Schoen AM and Wynn SG (Eds). Complimentary and Alternative Veterinary Medicine: Principles and Practice. Mosby, St. Louis 1998;53-69.

16 Sackman JE. Geriatrics: Pain and its management. Vet Clin N Am Sm Anim Prac 1997;27(6):1487-504.

17 Lee D, Papich M, Hardie EM. Pharmacokinetic distribution of transdermal fentanyl in cats. Am J Vet Res 1999: in press.

18 Pascoe P. Control of postoperative pain in animals receiving inhalant anesthetics: In: Short CE, Van Poznak A (Eds). Animal Pain. Churchill Livingstone, New York 1992:348-52.

19 Slingsby LS, Waterman-Pearson AE. Comparison of pethidine, buprenorphine and ketoprofen for postoperative analgesia after ovariohysterectomy in the cat. Vet Rec 1998;143:185-9.

20 Rainsford KD, Skerry TM, Chindemi P, Delaney K. Effects of the NSAIDs meloxicam and indomethacin on cartilage proteoglycan synthesis and joint responses to calcium pyrophosphate crystals in dogs. Vet Res Communications 1999;23:101-3.

9

PRACTICAL ANALGESIC TREATMENT IN EXOTIC ANIMAL SPECIES

Sharon Redrobe, BSc(Hons) BVetMed CertLAS MRCVS,
Bristol Zoo Gardens, Clifton, Bristol, UK

Introduction

Analgesia is often not considered for exotic animal species. This may be because of unfamiliarity with the signs or perception of pain in these species, the lack of published effective analgesic regimes or the misconception that analgesia may harm the animal. This is not a humane approach. Animals in pain will reduce their food and water intake and suffer from stress related disorders. Inadequate analgesia can seriously compromise post-operative recovery. Always give the animal the benefit of the doubt if pain is suspected. Analgesics administered appropriately and at the correct dose will not harm the animal.

The recognition of pain or discomfort in exotic animals can be difficult to perceive. Examples of signs of pain in these animals are given in Table 1. Some species have strong behavioural responses that hide signs of pain. The 'immobility' response of rabbits to manual restraint, especially when scruffed and restrained in dorsal recumbency, has often been suggested to be a form of 'anaesthesia' and analgesia. However, it has been reported that, although the animal may not show a withdrawal response to a painful stimulus, the physiological changes in heart rate and respiratory rate indicate distress [1]. This method should not be used therefore as a substitute for analgesia, sedation or general anaesthesia.

Birds are able to mask signs of illness until the late stage of disease when they rapidly decompensate. This can make them appear to be high-risk anaesthetic subjects as the patient may be more compromised than anticipated. A thorough pre-anaesthetic check is therefore vital in these patients, including blood biochemistry, haematology and radiography as well as a clinical examination to adequately assess the avian patient. Furthermore, birds can suppress severe arthritis pain when placed in novel pens or during egg laying behaviour [2]. However, this strong behavioural response should not preclude the routine use of analgesia in avian patients when procedures anticipated to produce pain are performed. A clinical examination, appropriate diagnostic techniques and supportive therapy must be used to assess and assist the avian patient during the peri-anaesthetic period. There are considerable species differences in the reaction to a painful stimulus. Many parrot species will react to pain by vocalising and showing a strong aversive response. Raptors and wild birds may become quiet and unresponsive when experiencing similar pain or discomfort.

The use of analgesia is still controversial in reptile medicine. It is difficult to assess whether a reptile is experiencing pain. Some lizards will not show a pedal withdrawal response when a digit is squeezed yet will show a strong aversive response to light touch. Some reptiles, especially snakes and lizards, may become more aggressive when experiencing pain whereas chelonia may become depressed. The 'freeze' behavioural response of the stressed reptile must not be overlooked when attempting to elicit a pain response. It is a curious anathema that although reptiles are undoubtedly able to feel pain, self-inflicted burns in captive reptiles are surprisingly common. If allowed direct access to the heat source, many reptiles will lie on the hot surface and sustain deep burns (even penetrating the coelomic membrane) without reacting to pain. However, as reptiles have anatomical nervous pathways that register noxious stimuli centrally via a three-tier pain control system [3], analgesia should be given for anticipated painful procedures.

Chronic conditions

Chronic painful conditions can occur in exotic pet species (see Table 2). Whilst every effort must be made to resolve the underlying condition, analgesia is used to manage the pain in order to optimise the quality of life of the animal. If it is not possible to provide

Table 1
Signs of pain

Small mammals	Reptiles	Birds
Aggression	Immobility	Immobility, collapse
Overgrooming	Anorexia	Increased aggression
Lack of grooming	Abnormal	Abnormal posture or locomotion
Inactivity	locomotion	Less 'talking' or singing
Hiding at back of cage	Posture	Less response to human if
Hunched posture	Increased	previously tame and interactive
Increased respiratory rate	aggression	Picking or plucking over painful area
Polydypsia	Dull	
Anorexia	colouration	
Hyperthermia, hypothermia		
Tooth grinding		
Self trauma over painful area		
Ferrets -vocalising,		
regurgitation,		
Salivation, seizures,		
vomiting		
(Note: vocalising is		
usually rare)		

adequate analgesia, euthanasia must be considered as a humane option. It may be useful to hospitalise the patient in the short term to assess response to analgesia. If a positive response to analgesia is obtained, the type of drug and route of administration should be determined that will provide adequate analgesia on a practical level. The options for the provision of home pain relief are restricted by the regulations concerning the use of opioids and the route of administration. Many small mammals will become fearful of repeated injections and so administration via this route is rarely a long-term solution. Tablets may be used to dose some species, for example, large lizards or ferrets, but are not easily administered to many small mammals, birds or reptiles. Oral liquids may be administered by syringe directly into the mouth, through the drinking water or in food.

Rats have been shown to 'self dose' by eating buprenorphine impregnated gelatine cubes to provide analgesia post-operatively. The long-term use of NSAIDs may be contraindicated in older animals suspected of renal dysfunction or because long term use may predispose the animal to gastro-intestinal or renal side effects. The use of flunixin meglumine has been associated with the development of renal failure in birds. This has been suggested to be due to the different renal anatomy and physiology of birds compared to mammals [4]. The renal anatomy of reptiles is similar to birds. It would be advisable therefore to carefully monitor the use of NSAIDs in birds and reptiles and restrict their use to the short term. However, these considerations must be weighed against the beneficial effects of analgesia to improve the quality of life in cases when a clinical cure is not possible. Suggested analgesics for long-term use are given in Table 3.

Table 2
Common chronic conditions

Condition	Species commonly affected
Dental disease	Rabbit, chinchilla, guinea pig
Pododermatitis	Rabbit, guinea pig, rat
Osteomyelitis	Rabbit, rodent, reptile
Arthritis	Rabbit, rat
Articular gout	Tortoise, budgerigar, canary

Local analgesia

Short-term local analgesia may be useful to enable stress-free examination of a painful area or the pain-free administration of substances into a vein. The local analgesic dose should be carefully calculated to avoid overdose should accidental systemic absorption occur; this is especially important in the smaller animals. Selected local anaesthetic agents are given in Table 4.

Local analgesia is useful to provide additional analgesia during surgical procedures; the incision site may be infiltrated with a short

Table 3

Analgesics suggested for long term use

Drug	Species
Meloxicam	Rabbit, rodent (bird, reptile)
Aspirin	Bird

acting local analgesic. This may result in some small mammals gnawing the site on recovery however, presumably due to the lack of sensation in that area. Surgery of the sinuses in birds appears to be particularly painful and associated with post-operative mortality if analgesia is not provided. Local analgesia may be directly administered to the sinus intra-operatively.

Peri-operative analgesia

A thorough clinical examination should be performed to ensure that the animal is free from clinical disease, especially with regard to respiratory and cardiovascular function. The patient should be weighed immediately before surgery to enable correct dosing and to assist in the assessment of pain after the procedure. Food and water intake should be measured pre operatively and changes in intake observed post-operatively used to assess post-operative pain. An intravenous or intraosseous catheter may be pre-placed for intra-operative and post-operative drug administration. The patient should be handled correctly to minimise trauma and stress.

Intra-operative analgesia

Intra-operative analgesia provides for a smoother plane of anaesthesia. This may be provided by the general anaesthetic agent itself or added to the general anaesthesia protocol. Inhalational agents may be used to induce or maintain general anaesthesia. Isoflurane is considered by many to be the agent of choice for exotic species for

Table 4

Local anaesthetic agents and indications for use

Local anaesthetic agent	Site of application/ route	Indications for use	Species
EMLA cream	Applied to skin	Applied to the skin prior to intravenous injection or catheter placement	Rabbit ear vein Rodent lateral tail vein
Bupivicaine	Local subcuticular infiltration	At surgical sites prior to incision	All species
Bupivicaine	Intra-articular injection	For the relief of articular pain	Birds (gout) Mammals Reptiles?
Lignocaine	Into sinus	Prior to surgery or debridement of the sinuses	Birds
Xylocaine or lignocaine	Applied to endotracheal tube or directly to larynx	To prevent laryngospasm during endotracheal intubation	Especially rabbit, ferret
	Epidural	To relieve post surgical pain, intra-operative pain for limb amputation, dystocia	Technique limited by size of species; technically possible in ferret, rabbit, guinea pig
Lidocaine	Infiltrate local area	For local analgesia	4-6 mg/kg total dose reptiles
Ophthaine	Eye	To facilitate catheterisation and flushing of nasolacrymal duct	Rabbit

many reasons: the rapid induction and recovery, greater cardio-vascular stability, and lower organ toxicity, when compared with halothane. Nitrous oxide is used in animals weighing more than 2 kg, where the second gas effects will accelerate the uptake of other inhaled agents. As this effect is limited in smaller species it is rarely used in exotic species. Nitrous oxide provides no analgesia.

Small mammals

Injectable agents commonly used to provide analgesia and sedation or general anaesthesia in exotic mammals are given in Table 5. Fentanyl/fluanisone (Hypnorm, Janssen) provides good sedation and analgesia in small mammals. It is very safe in small mammals and is the drug of choice for restraint for minor procedures such as radiography or dental inspection. It can be given by the intravenous, intramuscular and intraperitoneal routes. The fentanyl component can be reversed with naloxone for reversal of the sedation and analgesia. Alternatively, it can be reversed with buprenorphine or butorphanol, allowing analgesia to be maintained. The disadvantages of this product include moderate respiratory depression, poor muscle relaxation, hypotension and bradycardia. Rabbits tend to be sedated and relaxed with this combination whereas guinea pigs tend to be quite tonic. Combination with a benzodiazepine (diazepam, midazolam) provides a good surgical general anaesthesia.

The use of ketamine alone is associated with an increase in muscular tone and variable analgesia. The intramuscular injection of ketamine is associated with pain and muscle damage in rabbits and rodents [5,6]. Levels of ketamine required for surgical anaesthesia produce severe respiratory depression in rodents. Combining ketamine with xylazine or medetomidine produces a safer general anaesthetic but is associated with hypotension. Atropine (0.5-1 mg/kg) or glycopyrrolate (0.1 mg/kg) may be used as a pre-medicant to control the excess salivation and bronchial secretions associated with this combination. Some rabbits produce an atropinase that shortens the effect of atropine to a few minutes; the atropine dose may be increased or repeated or the alternative glycopyrrolate used instead. However, the secretions may be made more viscous and thus more likely to block the small airways or endotracheal tubes of the smaller exotic animals. The sedative drug of choice for rabbits is the compound fentanyl/j158 fluanisone (Hypnorm, Janssen). This provides profound analgesia lasting up to 180 minutes [7]. The cardiovascular and respiratory parameters are less affected than with other common sedative combinations. Rapid reversal of the sedation and respiratory depression of fentanyl is achieved rapidly by naloxone. If the sedative effects are reversed with buprenorphine, combined analgesia is provided for 420 minutes yet the respiratory depression is reversed allowing the arterial pH, pCO_2 and pO_2 to return to pre-general anaesthetic levels [7].

Medetomidine can be used as chemical restraint for minor procedures in ferrets. The addition of ketamine or butorphanol increases the degree of analgesia provided without increasing the recumbency time [8]. Atipamezole may be used to reverse the medetomidine although, if medetomidine alone is used, this will then leave the ferret without analgesia. A longer period of analgesia, lasting up to 80 minutes, is associated with the general anaesthetic combination xylazine, butorphanol and ketamine than with combinations substituting xylazine for acetylpromazine or diazepam [9]. Agents commonly used to provide analgesia and sedation or general anaesthesia in the ferret are given in Table 6.

Birds

Agents commonly used to provide analgesia and sedation or general anaesthesia in birds are given in Table 7. Ketamine alone does not provide adequate analgesia for major surgical procedures. The pattern of respiration should be stable during anaesthesia. A change in the pattern, especially in the depth of respiration (from shallow to deep) may indicate that the bird's plane of anaesthesia is lightening or the bird is feeling pain. As an aid to the assessment of pain, the heart rate is dramatically effective. It is not uncommon for a cockatiel, on feeling pain, to increase its heart rate from 300 bpm to over 700 bpm [10].

Reptiles

Agents commonly used to provide sedation or general anaesthesia in reptiles are given in Table 8. Neuromuscular blocking agents are often used to chemically restrain reptiles. It must be remembered that these agents offer no analgesia. They should not be used as a substitute for analgesia or general anaesthesia in the performance of surgical procedures. Hypothermia has been recommended as a method of restraint; this also offers no analgesia and may compromise the immune system. Therefore, the use of neuromuscular blocking agents or hypothermia for the performance of painful procedures should be considered ethically unacceptable. Few studies have been conducted to investigate the analgesic component of the commonly used anaesthetic agents. It is to some extent assumed that following administration of an anaesthetic agent, when the reptile no longer reacts to a noxious stimulus, then a surgical plane of general anaesthesia has been achieved and that analgesia is also provided. Many reptiles become apnoeic once a state of general anaesthesia is achieved and IPPV is routine.

There are few studies detailing the depth of anaesthesia or how to assess this in reptiles. It is common for a reptile to have a long period of recovery from anaesthesia. It may be, therefore, that reptiles are often maintained at a deep plane of general anaesthesia in order to maintain immobility and that the addition of analgesia routinely to the anaesthetic regimes may result in faster recoveries. More research into this area is needed.

Reversal agents for the sedative and general anaesthetic combinations noted in Tables 5-8 are given in Table 9.

Post-operative care

Inadequate analgesia can seriously compromise post-operative recovery. Prolonged recovery may lead to muscular injury, damage to eyes, skin soiling, prolonged inappetence, hypothermia and eventually death. The animal should be monitored for signs of pain until full

Table 5

Injectable agents for sedation and general anaesthesia in mammals

Drug	Species (dosage in mg per kg bodyweight, unless otherwise indicated)				Duration of anaesthesia
	Mouse	Rat	Guinea pig/ chinchilla	Rabbit	
Fentanyl + fluanisone	0.2-0.5 ml i.m. or 0.3-0.6	As mouse	0.5 – 1.0 ml i.m.	0.2- 0.4 ml i.m.	Sedation only 30-45 min
Fentanyl / fluanisone + diazepam	0.4 ml/kg + 5	0,3 ml/kg + 2.5	1 ml/kg + 2.5	0.3 ml/kg i.m. + 2 i.v.	45-60 min
Fentanyl / fluanisone + midazolam	10 ml/kg solution**	2.7 ml/kg solution**	8 ml/kg solution**	0.3 ml/kg i/m + 0.5-1 i/v	45-60 min
Ketamine/ medeto- midine	200 + 0.5	90 + 0.5	40 + 0.5	35 i.m. + 0.5 i.m.	20-30 min
Propofol	26 i.v.	10 i.v.	-	10 i.v.	5 min

All doses intraperitoneal route unless otherwise stated

i.m. = intramuscularly

i.v. = intravenously

*   Fentanyl + fluanisone as Hypnorm (Janssen Pharmaceuticals)

**   prepare as one part fentanyl + fluanisone, 2 parts water, one part midazolam

Table 6
General anaesthetic and analgesic combinations in the ferret

Drug(s)	Doses (mg/kg)
Diazepam – butorphanol – ketamine	3 - 0.2 - 15
Acetylpromazine – butorphanol – ketamine	0.1- 0.2 - 15
Xylazine – butorphanol - ketamine	2 - 0.2 - 15
Tiletamine+zolazepam (Zoletil, Tetazol) – xylazine – butorphanol	1.5 - 1.5 - 0.2
Medetomidine-ketamine	0.1 - 0.8

Table 7
Injectable agents for sedation and general anaesthesia in birds

Anaesthetic	Dosage (mg/ kg)	Comments
Ketamine	20 – 50 s.c., i.m., i.v.	Smaller species require a higher dose rate than larger birds
Ketamine + diazepam/ midazolam	25 K+ 2.5 D i.m. 20 K + 0.5-1.5 D i.m. 25 K + 1 – 2 D or 0.2 Mid s.c., i.m.	20-30 min general anaesthesia
Ketamine/ medetomidine	Raptors 3-5 K/ 50-100 (µg/kg M i.m. Psittacines 3-7 K/ 75-150 (µg/kg M i.m.	1.5 – 2 mg/kg ketamine + 60 – 85 µg/kg medetomidine i.m. (reversed by atipamazole 250 – 380g/kg i.m.)
Ketamine/ xylazine	4.4 xylazine + 2.2 xylazine i.v.	Xylazine is reversed by yohimbine 0.1 mg, or atipamezole 250 – 380 g/kg i.m.
Propofol	3-5 i.v.	Short acting; care with transfer to gaseous anaesthetic

Table 8
Injectable agents for sedation and general anaesthesia in reptiles

Drug	Dosage mg/kg				Duration of action
	Ch	S	L	Cr	
Tiletamine HCl/ Zolazepam (Zoletil/Telazol)	3-10	10-30	10-25	1-2	i.m. induction 5-20 min; Recovery 2-10 hours
Ketamine	3-60	20-60	25-60	12-25	Lower doses used for sedation Recovery may take hours Poor muscle relaxation
Diazepam Acepromazine Propofol	0.37 – 0.5 i.m. 0.1–0.5 i.m. 10–15 i.v.				1 h prior to induction 30 sec. to act, 30-40 min duration
Alphadalone/ alphaxolone (Saffan)	9–12 i.v., i.m.				Variable response in chelonia

Ch = chelonia
S= snake
L = lizard
Cr = crocodilian

Table 9
Reversal agents for sedative and general anaesthetic combinations

Reversal agent	Drug reversed	Dosage and route
Atipamazole	Any combination using medetomidine or xylazine	1 mg/kg i.m., i.p., s.c., i.v.
Buprenorphine	Any combination using hypnorm	see analgesia Table i.m., i.p., s.c., i.v.
Butorphanol	Any combination using hypnorm	see analgesia Table i.m., i.p., s.c., i.v
Flumazenil	Benzodiazepine	0.1 mg/kg

recovery is noted. In general, the animal is recovered individually in a quiet, dimly lit area. The recovery area should be the correct temperature for the species. This is especially important for reptiles that need to be maintained within their preferred optimum temperature range (Table 10). The animal's core temperature must be monitored until it has recovered fully. Animals in pain will reduce their food and water intake and so inadequate analgesia can seriously compromise post-operative recovery in small mammals and birds that develop hypoglycaemia relatively quickly. Most reptiles are more able to withstand a period of anorexia post-operatively, but dehydration in these species predisposes them to visceral gout that may be fatal. Fluids (including glucose) may be administered if the animal does not begin eating and drinking within a reasonable period of time for the species. Analgesia is administered routinely after a procedure that may be painful or if assessment on recovery indicates pain.

Table 10

Normal temperature ranges for selected reptile species

Reptile	Environmental temperature range (°C)
Boa constrictor *Boa constrictor*	25-30
Cornsnake *Elaphe guttata*	25-30
Day gecko *Phelsuma cepediana*	23-30
Garter snake *Thamnophis* sp.	22-26
Green iguana *Iguana iguana*	26-40
Leopard gecko *Eublepharus macularius*	23-30
Royal python *Python regius*	25-30
Red eared terrapin *Trachemys scripta elegans*	20-30
Mediterranean (spur thighed) tortoise *Testudo graeca*	20-35

Rodents

Crieria of weight loss and food and water consumption changes are sensitive indicators of post-operative pain. Simple behavioural assessment may not be as helpful in assessing pain. A single, intra-operative dose of a NSAID is often sufficient analgesia after major surgery based on these criteria. The critical period for analgesic use is in the first 6-12 hours post-operatively for rats and mice.

Rabbits

Good peri-operative care, especially with regard to pain management, is vital for the success of the procedure. Rabbits in pain become anorexic and develop ileus that will require specific therapy, namely, gastrointestinal tract motility enhancers as well as analgesia, or the condition may be fatal. This sequel is a common cause of post-operative death in (non-analgesed) pet rabbits.

Characteristics of selected analgesics in birds

Butorphanol acts at μ- and κ-receptors. In budgerigars, 3 - 4 mg/kg butorphanol did not affect respiratory rate or heart rate yet led to reduced motor control [11]. Flunixin meglumine at 10 mg/kg had no effect on heart rate in budgerigars [11], motor control was normal but regurgitation occurred within 2 - 5 mins in 5/6 birds and tenesmus was also seen. Flunixin meglumine has been shown to cause renal damage in birds due to their different structural anatomy and renal haemodynamics from mammals [4]. Birds may show pain by vocalising, lack of vocalising (especially the speaking birds), biting at painful area, slow recovery from anaesthesia or even death on recovery as the painful stimulus is perceived. In cases of suspected spinal cord damage, one must assess pain perception as a lack of this function, which indicates a poor prognosis. Limb withdrawal alone does not require an intact spinal cord as this can occur as a segmental reflex; other signs of pain are vocalisation, or looking towards the affected point.

Table 11

Analgesic agents in exotic species (many of these doses are anecdotal and may not be licensed for the species)

Drug	Dosage (mg/kg) and route (s.c. unless otherwise stated)			
	Small mammal e.g. rat	Larger mammal e.g. rabbit, badger	Bird	Reptile
Buprenorphine	0.05-0.1	0.01-0.05	0.02 i.m.	Not established
Butorphanol	1-5	0.1-0.5	3 i.m.	Not established
Carprofen	5	1-5	5 – 10	5
Ketoprofen		5 i.m.	5 - 10 i.m.	
Morphine	2-5 s.c. q2-4h	2-5 s.c., i.m. q4h	Not established	Not established
Meloxicam	0.2	0.1-0.2	0.2	0.2

Summary

Although a wealth of data exists for small mammal analgesic protocols, less is available for birds and least for reptiles. Nevertheless, by appreciating that the anatomy and physiology of these animals indicate that they have the capacity to feel pain, analgesia should be provided in circumstances anticipated to cause pain. Knowledge of the species-type reaction to pain should assist the clinician in assessing the effect and requirement for continued analgesia. The practice of humane veterinary medicine must include the appropriate use of analgesia; the practice of exotic animal medicine is no exception.

References

1 Danneman PJ, White WJ, Marshall WK, Lang CM. An evaluation of analgesia associated with the immobility response in laboratory rabbits. Lab Anim Sci 1988;38(1):51-7.

2 Gentle MJ, Corr SA. Endogenous analgesia in the chicken. Neurosci Lett 1995;210(3):211-4.

3 Ten Donkelaar HJ, de Boer-van Huizen R. A possible pain control system in a non-mammalian vertebrate (a lizard, Gekko gecko). Neurosci Lett 1987;83(1-2):65-70.

4 Klein PN, Charmatz K, Langenberg J. The effect of flunixin meglumine on the renal function in Northern bobwhite (Coliinus virginianus): an avian model. Proc Am Assoc Zoo Vet 1994:128-31.

5 Beyers T, Richardson JA, Prince MD. Axonal degeneration and self-mutilation as a complication of intramuscular ketamine and xylazine in rabbits. Lab Anim Sci 1991;41:519-20.

6 Smiler KL, Stein S, Hrapkiewitz K, Hiben JR. Tissue response to intramuscular and intraperitoneal injection of ketamine and xylazine in rats. Lab Anim Sci 1990;40:60- 4.

7 Flecknell PA, Liles JH, Wootton R. Reversal of fentanyl/ fluanisone neuroleptanalgesia in the rabbit using mixed agonist/ antagonist opioids. Lab Anim 1989 23;23(2):147-55.

8 Ko JC, Heaton-Jones TG, Nicklin CF. Evaluation of the sedative and cardiorespiratory effects of medetomidine, medetomidine– butorphanol, medetomidine–ketamine, and medetomidine– butorphanol – ketamine in ferrets. J Am Anim Hosp Assoc 1997;33(5):438-48.

9 Ko JC, Smith TA, Kuo WC, Nicklin CF. Comparison of anaesthetic and cardiorespiratory effects of diazepam–butorphanol– ketamine, acepromazine–butorphanol– ketamine, and xylazine– butorphanol-ketamine in ferrets. J Am Anim Hosp Assoc 1998;34(5):407-16.

10 Lawton MPC. Anesthesia. In: Manual of Psittacine Birds. P.H. Beynon, N.A. Forbes, M.P.C. Lawton (Eds). BSAVA, Cheltenham 1996.

11 Bauk L. Analgesics in avian medicine. In: Proceeding of the Association of Avian Veterinarians Annual Conference, AAV, Lake Worth, 1990:239-44.

10

PRACTICAL ANALGESIC TREATMENT IN HORSES

Urs Schatzmann, DVM, PhD, DipECVA, Klinik für Nutztiere und Pferde der Universität Bern, Bern, Switzerland

Introduction

Horses with symptoms of severe pain must have been observed over many centuries. It is historically reported that pain has been treated for more than 3000 years with a variety of different substances and vegetable extracts such as poppy, hemp, alcohol, mandrake root, henbane seed, lettuce, willow bark.

Chronic pain of medium or lower intensity, as expressed by different grades of lameness, back pain under the saddle or chronic pain originating from internal diseases was not, and is still not considered as a problem in many regions of the world. Surgical interference in horses has been described and illustrated for hundreds of years and it must be assumed that most interventions (i.e. castrations, wound therapies, trephining of the sinus, neurectomies) were performed in the mechanically immobilised horse without adequate analgesia. However, today, there is wide acceptance in developed countries that painful interventions must be performed only under general or local anaesthesia, and treatment of acute or chronic pain in horses is also essential on humane grounds.

Pain in horses

Modern usage and many common diseases of horses provoke, possibly more than in other domestic animals, conditions of pain and inflammation. Surgical interference is followed by postoperative pain. Inflammation is a common sign of injured body tissues in relation to work, accidents and age, irrespective of the cause of the injury. The nature of the work of the horse, its weight, size and speed, cause sprains and strains, failure of ligaments, tendons, joints and bone, which may lead to temporary or permanent disability. The horse is, in contrast to other mammals, more sensitive to acute abdominal disorders causing pain and inflammation and often shows signs of acute pain and distress.

Signs of pain

The conscious horse expresses pain in many ways, depending on its localisation, severity and the horse's temperament. 'Cold-blooded' draught horses seem to be less sensitive to painful stimuli compared to 'warmbloods' and thoroughbreds, although this could well be a difference in behavioural response only. In addition, wide individual variation within the same breed appears to exist.

Although acute abdominal pain (colic) is easy to detect, recognition of acute or chronic pain originating from muscles, joints, bones and tendons is sometimes difficult and requires a profound knowledge of the normal behaviour of a horse. Mainly due to their size and strength, horses efficiently resist surgical stimuli without adequate analgesic regimes as long as they are not mechanically immobilised. Painful interventions should, based upon practical as well as ethical grounds, be performed with adequate sedation and analgesia only.

General and specific signs of pain in horses are listed in Table 1.

A horse with acute and severe pain has a unique facial expression. The normal movement of the ears is abolished, the eyes appear smaller with dilatated pupils and the facial expression is anxious and the nostrils are flared. Increased body temperature, arterial blood pressure, respiratory and heart rate and sometimes profuse sweating are the result of activation of the sympathicoadrenal system. Acute visceral pain, originating from distention or inflammation within the gastrointestinal tract, provokes clearly visible signs of increased locomotor activity with intermittent periods of lateral or dorsal recumbency in an attempt to relieve traction on the mesentery and

Table 1
Signs and origin of pain in horses

Acute pain

general: change in facial expression, anxious appearance, flared nostrils, wide open eyes, excessive sweating, not eating, increased pulse and respiratory rate

specific abdominal pain
gastric or mesenteric disorders (colic)

increase in locomotor activity,
kicking, looking backwards, scraping,
change in body position, restless up to panicking,
up and down, lying on the back
severe cases: dullness

specific locomotor system
laminitis, fractures, excessive
wounds, peri- or post-operative pain,
myositis, tetanus

high grade lameness,
increase in body temperature,
difficulties to stand or to get up,
reluctant to move or to bend the neck

Chronic pain

intraabdominal or
intrathoracic origin
change in appetite, weight loss,
change in appearance of the coat,
dull appearance,
change in personality or attitude

locomotor system

chronic lameness,
loss of gait and performance,
change in posture,
limbs in unusual position,
difficulties under the saddle
(back pain)

related viscera. The horse may be looking backwards and scrapes the floor or ground. Severe pain can provoke panic with self-mutilation. Dullness in the later stages of acute abdominal disorders is, however, more indicative of endotoxemia and not necessarily pain related.

Severe acute pain symptoms of peripheral origin are generally based on a clearly defined clinical problem. In the horse an inflammatory process within the hoof is a commonly diagnosed problem with most severe pain symptoms. Laminitis, hoof abscesses and puncture wounds provoke an acute and severe pain response. Myositis of large muscle masses, fractures and extensive wounds involving tendons, joints and periostal structures are also a common source of severe pain. Such horses are often reluctant to move, show high-grade lameness and often remain recumbent (sternal or lateral) and rise only with considerable difficulty.

All these symptoms require immediate pain relief. The recognition and the evaluation of pain symptoms of a lower degree during work is much more difficult. In the stable or in the fields, horses may show varying degrees of lameness at the walk or trot, and they may try to place the limbs in unusual positions to alleviate pain when not mobile. Sometimes quite unusual positions are observed. The best known is the alternating and frequent weight shifting to alleviate pressure on the diseased navicular area. In sporting disciplines, horses perform quite normally with lower degrees of lameness, and symptoms of pain are very discrete and visible only to the experienced horseman. Performance under the saddle or in harness is therefore a poor and insufficient indicator of equine welfare.

Pain originating from the cervical, thoracic or lumbar vertebrae is even more difficult to see and locate, because lameness is not a predominant symptom.

The recognition and evaluation of chronic pain originating from internal diseases can also be difficult. We can assume that the normal behaviour of a horse with chronic pain is altered to a greater or lesser degree. Sometimes, changes in temperament and attitude are observed. Loss of appetite and weight loss, together with alterations in attitude and appearance and sometimes mild signs of colic may suggest that horses are suffering from pain. The origin of this pain must be considered to be mainly in the abdominal or thoracic cavity.

Principles and ethics of pain treatment

Pain is a natural defence mechanism against tissue injury and should lead to successful tissue healing. In the horse as in other species, pain also has, in some situations, a certain protective function to prevent further damage, i.e. bone fissures are protected from fracturing; affected areas need immobilisation for better healing. In these rare cases, treatment of pain is therefore contraindicated. In most cases, however, a pain producing process itself causes further injury. This occurs mainly in colic cases, in the postoperative period after painful surgical interventions and whenever excessive pain symptoms (irrespective of their origin) are present. Hence it is appropriate to intervene with analgesic and anti-inflammatory medication. All efforts should be directed to resolving the underlying problem: a horse with colic may need surgery, abscesses need drainage, chronically lame horses must be withdrawn from sport.

As stated above, many horses with minor pain symptoms originating from chronic degenerative processes in the locomotor system are worked regularly and may also perform successfully in competitions. Although it could be stated that these animals need anti-inflammatory medication to treat the pain, the national and international federations as well as many animal protection laws do not allow medication of these horses, mainly to give the same chances to all competitors and to determine the breeding potential not only on the basis of performance but also of soundness.

Is it ethically acceptable to control chronic inflammation and pain on a regular basis for daily pleasure work? Is it appropriate to administer 'painkillers' to a chronically lame horse out in pasture or can we assume that a low-grade lameness does not require medication? It is our opinion that a visibly lame horse should not be worked and that regular medication for this purpose should be avoided. The application of an anti-inflammatory or analgesic medication in show- or racehorses with degenerating diseases in the locomotor system is an unethical act. A clearly visible chronic lameness can be tolerated without medication when the horse is not worked and kept at pasture. The pain sensation is, in these cases, judged to be tolerable. For horses in severe pain with no chances for improvement, euthanasia must be considered.

Pain measurement and determination

Due to the wide variety of biochemical, physiological and behavioural parameters which change in horses with pain, adequate statistical analyses to determine the degree of pain and the requirement for analgesic medication are not readily available. Although a complex series of sympathetic, hormonal and metabolic changes, that occur in response to a noxious stimulus can be measured, these parameters are considered as a stress response and are not pain specific [1]. In discussion of different clinical signs of pain, using a pain scoring system, Zierz and Wintzer [2] showed a clear relationship between the adrenalin and noradrenalin concentration in blood and the degree of acute pain symptoms.

To assess the effectiveness of analgesics (and sedatives) in the horse, different pain models varying from the cutaneous stimulus with a prick of a needle to the determination of evoked potentials have been described [3]. Most of these tests are based on the alteration of the pain threshold to an increasing noxious stimulus. Invasive models include dental dolorimetry, an implanted heat element and distensible balloons implanted in the caecum or located in the stomach. Non-invasive methods include a light beam focused on the skin, a heat element applied to the skin, electric stimulation or a pressure device applied to the metacarpus. These tests allowed the determination of the analgesic activity and the duration of effect of drugs including α2-agonists, analgesics and some NSAIDs. The effect of flunixin meglumine and carprofen on threshold pressure with a distensible balloon introduced in the stomach is illustrated in Fig. 1. It can be demonstrated that both drugs exert a strong effect on visceral pain perception.

The analgesic effect of detomidine, romifidine and xylazine, as determined by the threshold current applied to the skin is shown in Figure 2.

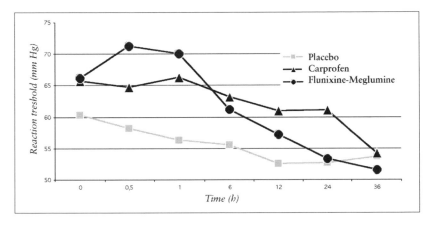

Figure 1 *Alterations in threshold pressure (balloon model in the stomach) under the influence of carprofen, flunixin and placebo (mean values, n = 6 horses).*

The effect of opioids such as butorphanol or l-methadone (in l-Polamidone) administered to increase analgesia and sedation provoked by an α2-agonist such as romifidine (or detomidine) can be measured with the electric current (Fig. 3) or pressure model.

The possibility of assessing pain perception through Electro-encephalography (EEG) is also under debate in the horse. The possibility of evaluating nociception under general anaesthesia has been discussed [4]. In awake horses the use of an EEG is too non-specific for assessment of pain perception.

Methods for treatment of pain

The different methods and drug groups are summarised in Table 2.

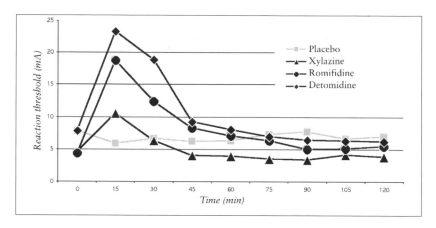

Figure 2 *Alterations in threshold current (electric current model) under the influence of xylazine, romifidine and detomidine (mean values, n = 6 horses).*

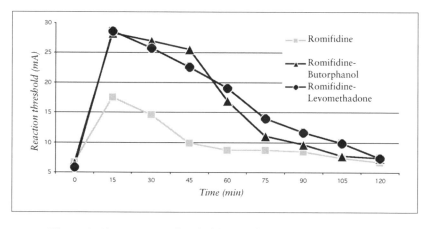

Figure 3 *Alterations in threshold current (electric current model) under the influence of romifidine alone and in combination with butorphanol or l-methadone (mean values, n = 6 horses).*

Table 2

Methods of controlling pain in horses

Direct pain effect (no effect on inflammation)	
	Narcotic analgesics
	α2-Agonists
	Local anaesthetics
Mainly on inflammation (followed by pain relief)	
	NSAIDs
	Corticosteroids
With no medication	Cold packs
	Nose twitch
	Acupuncture analgesia
	Neurectomies

Physical methods

Of the various physical methods that might be used to control pain, cold is perhaps the most generally used in acute stages of swellings in the distal limb, originating from tendinitis, bruises or inflammation of joints. Regular hosing, standing in cold water or applying ice packs are traditional forms of alleviating acute local pain and swelling. Topically applied aerosol sprays that cause surface cooling may be used for pain-free insertion of large bore catheters or injection needles through the skin.

Acupuncture

According to a number of reports, acupuncture treatment also provides analgesia in the horse [5]. It appears to be a form of treatment that should be seriously considered for the treatment of chronic pain. It is not a rapid method and involves repeated treatments over a period of time. Interesting studies have shown beneficial effects in cases of laminitis and chronic back pain [5, 6]. Acupuncture therapy is restricted to specialists with training and experience. No experience, however, is needed for a daily used variant of acupuncture: the horse twitch.

The twitch procedure is used to immobilise horses and, although no scientific results are available, it is obvious that the pain threshold is increased. Endorphin systems are probably involved in the effectiveness since its action is blocked by naloxone and increased β-endorphin levels have been measured [7].

Local, regional and spinal anaesthesia
Local, perineural or epidural infiltrations of local anaesthetics are extensively used in the sedated horse mainly for wound repair. Lidocaine is still the most widely used agent.

Local anaesthetics have been administered in the epidural space for many years to provoke analgesia in the perianal region. Larger doses affect the motor nerves of the hind limbs and provoke paralysis and are therefore contraindicated. In recent years α2-agonists and opioids, administered by caudal epidural injection have shown to provide pain relief with dermatomal spread up to the thoraco-lumbar region. However, the method is not yet routinely used for postoperative or chronic pain control in the horse.

Neurectomy
The transection of a peripheral nerve is a palliative treatment used mainly to relieve pain originating from the navicular area. Historically, all nerves in the front and hind limbs have been transected, but the methods have fallen into disuse. Today only the neurectomy of the distal digital nerves below the fetlock joint is performed. Neurectomised horses should not compete and should not be used for hard work, since the underlying disease is not influenced by the surgery. Normally, the sensation is restored within one year due to the regrowth of the nerve fibres.

Systemic pain medication
Non-steroidal anti-inflammatory drugs (NSAIDs)
The non-steroidal anti-inflammatory drugs are among the most widely used substances in equine medicine and are used in all conditions presenting pain, inflammation and fever. The main substances used are listed in Table 3.

Table 3

Commonly used NSAIDs

	Suggested dose	Elimination half life (h)
Salicylates	20 mg/kg orally	5 - 7
Flunixin meglumine	1.1 mg/kg	1.6
Naproxen	5 mg/kg	4
Meclofenamic acid	2.2 mg/kg	0.9
Phenylbutazone	4 - 8 mg/kg	3.5 - 8
Carprofen	0.7 mg/kg	18
Metamizole	25 mg/kg	5
Ketoprofen	1.1 mg/kg	1.5
Diclofenac	0.5 mg/kg	6 – 8
Vedaprofen	1 mg/kg orally	0.7 – 2.2
N-Butylscopolamine	0.3 mg/kg (only spasmolytic activity)	

Some of the products may not be available in different countries because of registration and legislation differences, and they have different trade names.

NSAIDs inhibit the cyclooxygenase enzyme, interrupt formation of thromboxane, prostacyclin and prostaglandin from arachidonic acid [8]. Recent research has also shown that some of the NSAIDs act on pain receptors in the central nervous system and block pain in the same manner as analgesic drugs such as morphine.

The use of the available NSAIDs in the horse, mainly in high doses and for longer periods, is not without toxicity. Deleterious effects, mainly related to phenylbutazone medications, have been well known for many years [8]. Toxic effects are visible in the intestinal tract with the danger of colitis and ulceration. A comparative study with ketoprofen, flunixin and phenylbutazone, administered in high doses for several days, produced evidence of stomach ulcers with all the three substances whereas the small and large intestines were affected mainly by phenylbutazone [9].

Potency and clinical use

All of the currently available NSAIDs alleviate pain and/or inflammation in the horse. It must be accepted that extreme pain, originating from the intestinal tract or from severe inflammation in the hoof (i.e. laminitis) cannot be abolished even with highest (and toxic) doses of any NSAID.

Depending on the origin of pain, extreme differences in potency exist. Laboratory animal studies, adapted for horses [8], revealed an order of potency for anti-inflammatory activity of:

Flunixin > Meclofenamic acid > Phenylbutazone > Ketoprofen > Naproxen > Salicylates.

This order is of questionable value. Depending on the origin of pain, extreme differences in potency exist. From clinical experience it is our view that phenylbutazone exerts a specific action on the locomotor system, especially when the hoof and the distal joints are involved, whereas flunixin and metamizole are preferable for use in visceral pain (colic). Clearly defined studies for comparison of effect and duration of all NSAIDs in different pain models do not exist. The choice of a medicament is therefore dependent on the personal preference and experience of the veterinary surgeon and, to a lesser extent, on marketing strategies of the pharmaceutical companies.

Salicylates

Clinical experience would suggest that salicylates have the weakest anti-inflammatory and analgesic activity of all NSAIDs and are rarely used for this reason in the horse. They are occasionally given to treat fever. Their anti-clotting action (5-10 mg/kg daily) is useful in treating conditions that involve damage of blood vessels and blood thrombi (mainly laminitis and thrombosis).

Flunixin meglumine

Flunixin meglumine is used in horses for inflammatory and painful conditions and is administerated either by the i.v., i.m. or oral route. It is specifically recommended as an analgesic in colic and for the treatment of endotoxic shock. It may, however, cause problems in the acurate diagnosis of colic due to its effectiveness and long duration of action. It is widely used clinically also for postoperative pain because of its low toxicity. The effect is difficult to assess. In colic pain it acts immediately and the effects are longer lasting than for metamizole. In orthopaedic cases it is not as effective as phenylbutazone.

Naproxen

Although it has been on the market for many years, naproxen is seldom used and it is not registered in many countries. The effect is comparable to phenylbutazone and it seems to by particularly effective in soft tissue inflammation [8].

Meclofenamic acid

Meclofenamic acid is available in some countries in the oral form. It has a slow onset of action and the effect is comparable to that of phenylbutazone. It seems to be particularly useful in acute and chronic laminitis and skeletal conditions. The toxic effects are similar to those of phenylbutazone.

Phenylbutazone

Phenylbutazone is the most extensively used NSAID in the horse for all common musculo-skeletal disorders and seems to have, in comparison with other NSAIDs, a most specific action in navicular disease, laminitis, osteoarthritis and other degenerative joint diseases. It is used in different formulations (injectable, powder, paste, and tablets). Unfortunately, it has been withdrawn from the EU market for legal reasons.

Although phenylbutazone has important acute toxic effects, low doses (0.2 g/100 kg per day) given for longer periods produced very few unwanted side effects in a large number of horses.

Carprofen

Carprofen is a relatively new and effective NSAID because of its long half-life in plasma [10]. It is only registered in a limited number of countries. The effect is comparable to flunixin with a longer action as demonstrated in visceral and peripheral pain models. Clinical experience showed less effect in musculo-skeletal disorders when compared to phenylbutazone.

Metamizole (Dipyrone®, Novaminsulfon®)

Dipyrone has analgesic, antipyretic and slight anti-inflammatory properties in the horse. It has spasmolytic activity and is therefore extensively used in colic therapy as the first choice medicament. The response is valuable and gives information about the severity of the underlying problem in the gastrointestinal tract. Metamizole does not have the potency of flunixin. In musculo-skeletal disorders the effect can be judged as insufficient when compared to other NSAIDs.

Ketoprofen

Ketoprofen does not appear to be substantially different from flunixine meglumine for clinical use in the horse. The maximum anti-inflammatory effects occur at 12 hours after administration and last for 24 hours. It produces fewer gastrointestinal lesions than phenylbutazone and is recommended for musculo-skeletal injuries, but it is less effective in acute joint inflammation than phenylbutazone.

Vedaprofen

Recently released in some EU countries, vedaprofen, a new NSAID from the arylpropionic acid class, is presented as an gel formulation for oral use in horses. It has been shown to be highly protein-bound and to accumulate in inflammatory exsudate. Experimental work performed in horses has shown that vedaprofen induced a significant inhibition of inflammatory swelling and an inhibition of migration of leukocytes into the exsudate. Although the mechanism behind these effects has not been fully elucidated, it is suggested that these properties can be considered favourable for clinical practice [11].

Diclofenac

Diclofenac is a well known NSAID in human medicine to be registered for horses in the near future. According to preliminary results it exerts a strong action in musculo-skeletal disorders with a duration comparable to phenylbutazone. Nothing is known yet about the toxicity.

Narcotic analgesics

Narcotic analgesics have long been used in the horse, particularly to control the acute pain of colic. Nearly all substances used in other mammals or in man have been associated with excitement and/or with unpredictable reactions in the horse (central nervous stimulation, increased locomotor activity, etc.) when given in effective doses. According to comparative analgesia tests for superficial, deep and visceral pain and from personal experience, only butorphanol showed analgesic activity as demonstrated in the visceral pain model [12]. Opioids are routinely co-administered with sedatives or tranquilizers (acepromazine, α2-agonists) to enhance the sedative and analgesic effect without showing adverse signs (Fig. 3).

As a sole drug, only butorphanol in a dosage of 0.1 mg/kg, administered i.v. or i.m. (the i.v. route is preferable), can be suggested for relief of colic pain in the horse. Pain relief, however, is better with N-butylscopolamine or α2-agonists also in colic.

Alpha-2 agonists

All three commercially available and registered α2-agonists [xylazine (Rompun®), romifidine, (Sedivet®) and detomidine (Domosedan®)] produce analgesia, sedation and a dramatic depression of activity in the central nervous system [4]. These products are clinically used worldwide to obtain profound sedation and for sedative premedication. They are also used in a mixture with ketamine and guaifenesine to maintain anaesthesia by infusion.

In comparison with NSAIDs and opioids, α2-agonists are the most effective analgesics for visceral as well as for somatic pain, as demonstrated in clinical practice and in pain models.

When used in equisedative doses the differences in analgesic effects are minimal and a duration of analgesia of about 45 minutes with a maximum effect of 15 min after administration can be expected (Fig. 2).

Equisedative dosages of the three available α2-agonists

Xylazine	1.1 mg/kg
Detomidine	20 µg/kg
Romifidine	80 µg/kg

Because of the short duration of analgesia and because of the strong sedative effect of these substances, pain management of longer duration (i.e. for postoperative pain, laminitis, myositis, joint or hoof infections) is not possible.

Combination of tranquilizers/sedatives with narcotic analgesics

Although opioids *per se* are of limited value in horse pain for the reason stated above, they exert a strong and measurable analgetic effect when combined with α2-agonists (Fig. 3) or acepromazine. The combination with l-polamidone (Polamivet®) has been used in German speaking countries for more than 30 years without any reported untoward side-effects. The simultaneous administration of butorphanol and α2-agonists has shown its efficacy in last years, mainly in the USA and in Great Britain. It would appear that no differences between butorphanol and l-polamidone are detectable. The mixtures not only improve analgesia but also deepen and stabilise the sedative effects of α2-agonists. They are judged to be the most effective analgesic and sedative medication in the horse.

Dosage

Romifidine	40 µg/kg		L-Methadone 100 µg/kg
Xylazine	0.5 mg/kg	+	or
Detomidine	10 µg/kg		Butorphanol 25 µg/kg

Corticosteroids

Corticosteroids possess potent anti-inflammatory activity also in the horse. In acute inflammation, the corticosteroids maintain the integrity of blood vessels and reduce oedema formation and limit the movement of white blood cells into injured tissues. In later stages of wound healing, corticosteroids reduce the proliferation of blood vessels and connective tissue, which decreases scar tissue production and slows the wound healing process. Administration of corticosteroids is therefore contra-indicated for post-operative pain treatment.

Local injections of corticosteroids into joints or into tendons relieve pain and inflammation and help return normal function. However, if the underlying damage is not corrected, continued use of the horse will only cause further detoriation. This is especially marked in the case of tendinitis. Injected joints initially show less pain and swelling than non-injected joints; however, production of normal bone and cartilage ceases and normal joint lubricating substances are reduced. Continued mechanical trauma results in destruction of joint surfaces, loss of joint function and can ultimately lead to permanent disability of the horse. The use of corticosteroids as 'painkillers' is therefore generally not indicated.

References

1 Taylor P.M. Stress responses to anaesthesia in horses. In: Short CE, van Poznak A (Eds). Animal Pain. Churchill Livingstone, New York 1992:322-5.

2 Zierz J, Wintzer HJ. Über den akuten Schmerz beim Pferd und eine Möglichkeit seiner objektiven Bestimmung. Tierärztl Prax 1996;24:108-12.

3 Matthews NS. A review of equine pain models. In: Short CE, van Poznak A. (Eds). Animal Pain. Churchill Livingstone, New York 1992:403-7.

4 Short CE, Kallfelz FA, Otto K, Otto B, Wallace R. The effects of an α2-adrenoreceptor against analgesia on the central nervous system in an equine model. In: Short CE, van Poznak A (Eds). Animal Pain. Churchill Livingstone, New York 1992:421-34.

5 Klide AM. Use of acupuncture for the control of chronic pain and for surgical anaesthesia. In: Short CE, van Poznak A (Eds). Animal Pain. Churchill Livingstone, New York 1992:249-57.

6   Bossut DFB, Page EH, Stromberg MW. Production of cutaneous analgesia by electroacupuncture in horses: Variations dependent on sex of subject and locus of stimulation. Am J Vet Res 1993; 45:620-5.

7   Lagerweij E, Nelis PC, Wiegant VM, van Ree JM. The twitch in horses: a variant of acupuncture. Science 1984;225:1172-4.

8   Lees P, Higgins AJ. Clinical pharmacology and therapeutic uses of non-steroidal anti-inflammatory drugs in the horse. Eq Vet J 1985;17:83-96.

9   MacAllister CG, Morgan SJ, Borne AT, Pollet RA. Comparison of adverse effects of phenylbutazone, flunixin meglumine, and ketoprofen in horses. J Am Vet Med Ass 1993;202:71-7.

10 Schatzmann U, Gugelmann M, von Cranach J, Ludwig BM, Rehm WF, Baumgartner T, Stauffer JL. Visceral and peripheral pain detection models in the horse, using flunixin and carprofen. In: Short CE, van Poznak A (Eds). Animal Pain. Churchill Livingstone, New York 1992:411-20.

11 Lees P, May SA, Hoeijmakers M, Coert A, Rens PV. A pharmacodynamic and pharmacokinetic study with vedaprofen in an equine model of acute nonimmune inflammation. J Vet Pharmacol Therap 1999;22:96-106.

12 Pippi NN, Lumb WV. Objective tests of analgesic drugs in ponies. Am J Vet Res 1979;40:1082-6.

INDEX